P.R.O.V.E.R.B.S. D.I.E.T. WELLNESS PLAN

My children, do not forget my teaching, but keep my commands in your heart, for they will prolong your life many years and bring you prosperity. [**Proverbs 3:1-2 NIV**]

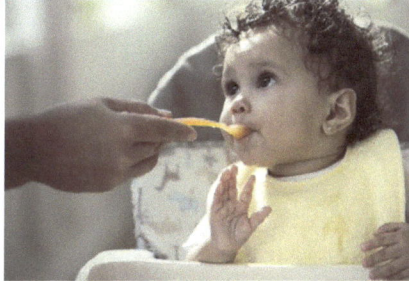

I0023239

Contents
Introduction of P.R.O.V.E.R.B.S. D.I.E.T. Wellness Plan
Step 1. **D**ecide to Stop (The Pain)
Step 2. **I**ncorporate (God's Pharmacy)
Step 3. **E**ducate by Sharing (God's Promise)
Step 4. **T**ransform to Fulfill (God's Purpose)

Disclaimer
Nothing written in this plan should serve as a replacement for medical care. Before undertaking any changes in diet or exercise consult your physician; especially, if you are currently on medication or under a doctor's care.

Acknowledgement
I am grateful to my loving and supporting family who shaped my life. Words cannot express my sincere love and gratitude. I am honored to have supportive friends and business partners whom I love, respect and admire. Special thanks to Rev. William A. Thurston, Ph.D. for providing content, support and ideas. Without you P.R.O.V.E.R.B.S. D.I.E.T Wellness Plan [PDWP] would not have been possible. A special thanks to Phyllis Nash, Jerome Hughes and Ian Coleman for being the first to believe in my vision of improving the health of the world through the P.R.O.V.E.R.B.S. D.I.E.T. book series. I thank God for his grace and mercy in allowing me to share this message with you.

This is a Gift From_____ **To**_____

Introduction

This will bring health to your body and nourishment to your bones. [Proverbs 3:8 NIV]

If, on opening these pages, you expect to find a magic bullet based on the advice to stop eating carbs or wheat to make all your problems disappear, you'll be disappointed. What are the two things that everyone is most consumed with multiple times per day? We are lifetime consumers driven by our insatiable **hunger** and **thirst**. In the United States we spend nearly $2 trillion on food, alcohol, water, other beverages and supplements each year. Every Monday, ten million people go on a diet, and yet we are more obese than ever. This leads us to spend over $2.5 trillion on healthcare, and we are still suffering and dying prematurely. P.R.O.V.E.R.B.S. D.I.E.T.: *Wellness Plan* [PDWP] exposes the truth of why we are under attack and dying physically, mentally, and spiritually. Currently, this problem is primarily in the US. As our Western influence spreads, we are headed towards a global health crisis. Whether your desire is to lose 150 lbs., 15 lbs. or avoid premature death, this plan holds the answer. PDWP is based on biblical principles, scientific evidence and validation from real people.

This plan is inspired from the book P.R.O.V.E.R.B.S. D.I.E.T.: *Wellness for Your Life's Purpose* [PD]. PD is a two-fold process of personal development with an innovative support system that equips you with the knowledge you need to save you and your family using 8 resources, 4 steps and 84 foods. It is an in-depth 84-day system with additional recipes, scriptures, supplements and tools to help you achieve wellness for your life's purpose. It provides a simple system that is easy to follow for life.

PDWP is designed to provide you with an introduction to the complete program. Before you commit to 84 days you have an opportunity to commit to just 4 weeks, which is 28 days. During this 28-day period you incorporate the 8 essential resources of P.R.O.V.E.R.B.S. and the 4 inter-related steps of D.I.E.T. to improve your health, increase energy, restore beauty, regain confidence, and lose unhealthy pounds.

The next few pages reveal the consequences of your choices and highlight the pain. It is our goal that you **d**ecide to stop the pain and **i**ncorporate God's Pharmacy, as well as **e**ducate others of God's Promise by sowing seeds of wellness to **t**ransform your life to fulfill God's Purpose.

(Step 1) = $\underline{\text{D}}$ecide + Incorporate + Educate + Transform

DECIDE TO STOP "THE PAIN"

Fast-forward to the year 2030: **more than 60% of adults in the United States are obese and close to 100% are overweight.** In 1980, just 5% of US children were obese. By 2012 the figure had reached 18%, but now, in 2030, **50% of children are obese, with a Body Mass Index (BMI) greater than 30.** During this same time young adults in their 20s are on waiting lists for liver transplants due to fatty liver disease. (When the body accumulates more fat than necessary, the liver and adipose tissue starts to store the excess amount and the accumulation of fat in the liver is known as fatty liver disease). Liver transplants were once common in older adults, individuals with cirrhosis, cancer patients or those with hepatitis, but are now performed on the youth and young adults. In this period almost half of the adult population is diabetic, and an unprecedented number of children under the age of ten are diagnosed with diabetes, reproductive cancers and heart disease. Kidney dialysis centers have become more popular than McDonald's, with dozens of centers in every major city, and even present in small towns.

The Year 2013

As shocking as all of this sounds, some experts predict that this might happen much sooner than 2030. To some extent it is already occurring right now. The health of the people in the US is failing and we have just a small window of time in which to turn this trend around before the impact is so deeply woven into our society that there will be no reversing it. "Diseases of Affluence" are on the point of exploding, and if we do not take action this country will be crushed into oblivion. Due to the modern day conveniences of living in a developed country, "Diseases of Affluence" impact the rich, poor and middle class. And even if you are underweight or at your ideal weight, you are still not immune to this disease, because **thin and normal weight individuals are developing pancreatic cancer, thyroid cancer, heart disease, diabetes and other diseases related to the affluent American lifestyle.** You can see extra weight and excess belly fat, but you can't see kidneys that are failing, congestive heart failure, a clogged artery, a compromised immune system, or toxicity of the liver.

The percentage of overweight individuals in this country is now a massive 69%, while 36% of individuals are clinically obese. Kidney dialysis centers, while not as popular as

McDonald's just yet, are already in every major city. Do you recall seeing even one of these growing up, let alone dozens in major cities?

Tragically, most American parents are completely oblivious to the fact that the biggest threat facing their family's future is what they put on their plates and inside their glasses. Unknowingly, you have been allowing your children, your husband, your wife and your family to dig a premature grave with the very fork you provide them. **It is a new phenomenon called "chewacide."** This is a catastrophic problem that will cause the premature death of more than 70-80% of people in the US; this is the new reality.

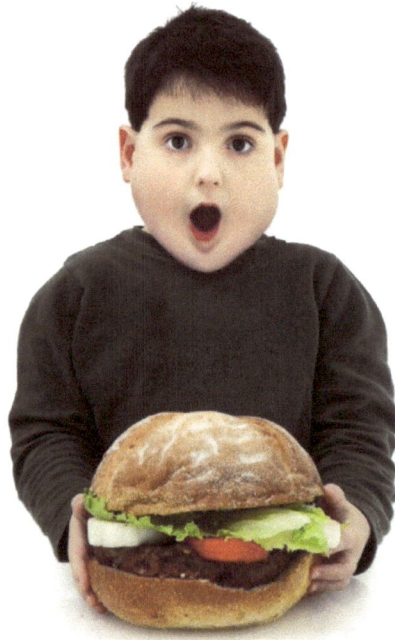

FOOD IS YOUR FAMILY'S LARGEST THREAT!

Fast foods, processed goods and items loaded with sugar are well-known for their negative impact on our health. While it is unmistakably clear that, in excess, these types of foods are lethal, the "true" modern seduction of our time is a silent deadly killer that's hard to identify because it is so deeply woven into the fabric of our culture. Instead of eating vegetables from the ground or fruit from trees, which was the original plan, we now consume artificially produced food made in laboratories (lab-made) in record quantities. Synthetic growth hormones are in the milk supply and in our meat. In addition to containing pesticides, fruits and vegetables have been manipulated and altered, creating a new species of lab-made food known as genetically modified organisms (GMOs). GMOs are proven to cause tumors, organ failure and a range of various health problems in animals. Neurotoxins such as monosodium glutamate (MSG) and aspartame are present in common everyday food consumed by our children and even our infants. These are toxic chemicals known to impact the brain and body. Companies spend millions of dollars on commercials aimed at children aired during cartoons and other shows enticing them with food containing these substances. Children develop the belief that these types of items improve their life.

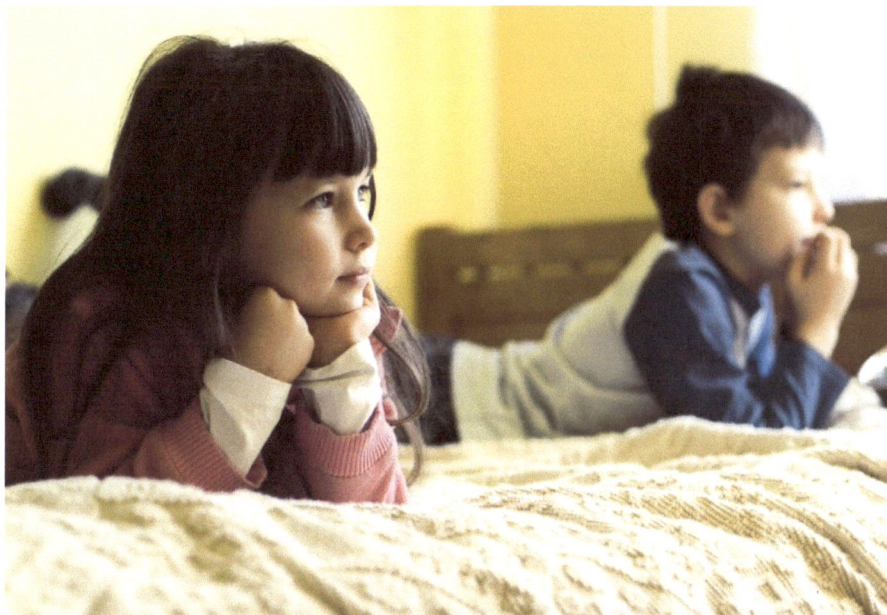

Our willingness to consume these items has created opportunities for companies to profit by billions of dollars, and the more toxic or processed the food the more profitable it is for big business. **The food that heals provides a 10%, or smaller, profit margin, while the food that kills provides a 90% or greater profit margin.** Between the food and medical industry, your poor health equals big business to the tune of trillions of dollars in revenue. As your family loses their health, big corporations are making billions of dollars off your pain. The system is broken. As a result, we are suffering consequences never experienced before by any other society.

An indicator of whether or not you or your child might be pre-diabetic is a condition known as acanthosis nigricans, which causes a darker, thick, velvety skin in body folds and creases. This can also signal other diseases, so check with your doctor. More often than not, however, it is a sign of insulin resistance. **Diabetes impacts 57 million Americans and is considered 95% preventable.** More than 70,000 people die each year from diabetes, but the majority of diabetics die from one of the risk factors associated with the disease, such as heart disease.

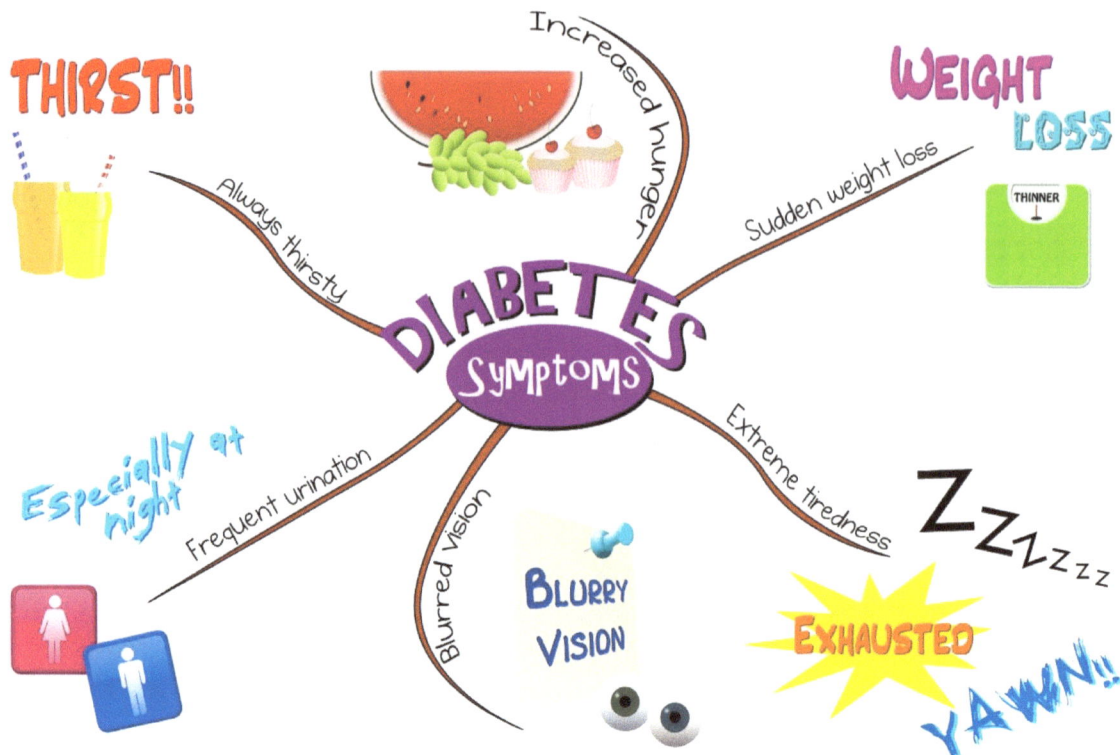

In the time it took you to read to this point, two dozen people or more will have experienced a heart attack or heart failure. Sadly, more than one-third of them will die. According to the Center for Disease Control (CDC), **heart disease killed 596,339 Americans in 2011**, and is the number one killer of both men and women in the US. To put this number in perspective, 123,000 people died in 2011 due to accidental injuries including automobile accidents. While this figure is horrific and by no means acceptable, the unsettling reality is that more than 4½ times more people succumb to death due to heart disease. The irony is that we spend most of our time worrying about accidents. **Heart disease impacts over 80 million Americans and is 90% preventable.**

In the United States, one of the wealthiest countries in the world, we suffer the consequences of the modern Western diet to a greater extent than any other country. Looking at a map of the world, you will see that virtually all chronic conditions like heart disease, diabetes, cancer and Alzheimer's are crowded into Western countries. Then there are countries, especially in Asia and Africa, where those diseases hardly show up at all. In fact, **the vicious cycle of these diseases are virtually nonexistent in more than 75% of the world.** There comes a point in our life when we stare death in the face and have to ask the question, "Is there any food or habit that is worth dying for?" When faced with our own mortality, the choice becomes that between premature death or dietary changes, exercise and/or recommended medical care.

Early screenings and preventative care are important for these diseases developed by our Western lifestyle. **Given the shocking statistic that 225,000 people in the US die each year from medical care** (including medication errors, unnecessary surgery, preventable hospital errors and hospital borne infections), avoiding disease through lifestyle modification certainly appears to be your best option. According to the World Health Organization (WHO), the US ranks 1st in the world for healthcare expenditures, but a dismal 37th for overall healthcare performance and 72nd for overall health out of 191 countries. The Commonwealth Fund ranked the US dead last in terms of quality of healthcare among similar countries. **For average life expectancy, the US ranks 37th of all the countries in the United Nations (UN),** but we still spend more money on healthcare than any other country.

Cancer is the second leading cause of death in the United States, claiming the lives of 575,313 in 2011 according to the CDC. **Cancer is 50-75% preventable and impacts 12 million Americans.** The reality is that one out of every three people we know will succumb to this awful disease. The consequence of cancer, which for many is death, drives people to extreme measures. For example, in the US, women who are identified with a gene linked to breast cancer are willing to remove their own and their daughter's breasts as a possible way to stop breast cancer from ever occurring. Whether we believe this procedure to be necessary or not, the reality is that breast cancer was virtually nonexistent in Japan until the 1950s, when they started adapting more of the Western lifestyle. **Women in the US are 20 times more likely than women in Kenya to develop breast cancer.**

Cancer will soon be the leading cause of death in the US. Lung cancer is the deadliest cancer, killing more people each year than colon cancer, breast cancer, pancreatic cancer and leukemia combined. **Lung cancer claimed the lives of 792,495 people between 2003 and 2007 in the US according to the National Cancer Institute (NCI).** It has been 47 years since the Food and Drug Administration (FDA) first required warning labels to be placed on cigarettes through the Federal Cigarette Labeling and Advertising Act of 1965, but it still kills more men and women than any other form of cancer.

One day you are told a low carbohydrate diet is the solution and the next you are told it is not. Do GMOs really cause reproductive cancer? Is wheat good or bad for me? Do I have wheat belly? Do I really have to buy organic food or is nonorganic food just as safe? Is a lack of vitamin D and dairy consumption really linked to prostate cancer? Olive oil is good one day and the next day it's not – who do you believe? Can excess animal protein really cause cancer? Will fish lower your risk of heart disease? If milk really prevents osteoporosis, why does the US have more hip fractures than non-milk drinking countries?

"If you can't convince them, confuse them." – Harry Truman

When you confuse a nation, a seed of complacency is sown. So there you have it: a passive society that willingly ingests substances like fake unnatural food, which yield death instead of life. This is the currency of deception. PDWP is designed to equip you with knowledge for navigating conflicting claims to develop your own diet for a long-lasting healthy life.

Is Your Life a Tragedy or a Testimony?

Disease is the diagnosis; it's the wakeup call that directs you to change your life, provided that the first symptom isn't death. But *"Dis-Ease"* is the slow process of aches, pains and warning signs you ignore until life-threatening disease, or even death itself, happens. There is no wealth without health. Steve Jobs had all the money in the world, but it couldn't save him. On February 28, 2013, I reached the age of 40. A few months prior to this milestone, I realized I had to make some changes.

Forty is a very significant number. Biblically, it is associated with tests and temptation. Life is about making decisions, which abort or advance life's purpose. **While the enemy uses temptations to destroy you, God permits tests and trials to develop you [Luke 4:1-3].** This is why so many people recognize 40 as the place where life begins because, until you are tested, there is no testimony. This period represents the time that God uses to prepare you for your life's purpose. For example, God used 40 days to transform the lives of Moses, Noah, David, and Jesus for their mission.

During the period of testing God is working within your spirit through your attitude and actions. God is working it out for the good by transforming adversity into advantage, including long-lasting health for advancing your life's purpose.

After fasting forty days and forty nights, he was hungry. [Matthew 4:2 NIV]

On the day Jonah entered the city, he shouted to the crowds: "Forty days from now Nineveh will be destroyed!" [Jonah 3:4 NLT] (The people repented in those 40 days and God spared the city.)

It also rained for 40 days and 40 nights when God wanted to cleanse the world and start over: *Seven days from now I will send rain on the earth for forty days and forty nights, and I will wipe from the face of the earth every living creature I have made.* [Genesis 7:4 NIV]

The Israelites spent 40 years in the wilderness: *Your children will be shepherds here for forty years, suffering for your unfaithfulness, until the last of your bodies lies in the wilderness. For forty years – one year for each of the forty days you explored the land – you will suffer for your sins and know what it is like to have me against you.* [Numbers 14:33-34 NIV]

From February 2012 through October 2012 I experienced a series of traumatic events that gave me the wakeup call I needed to take my health seriously. One of them included a reaction to an artificial chemical (found in food, drinks and gum) that left me with a bout of insomnia, depression and anxiety that lasted nine days. During this period, I got a total of 30 minutes of sleep. After sending my son a text instructing him on what to do if something happened to me, I went on a total detox program to get rid of the toxins and transform my health.

Food can be your best friend and worst enemy at the same time, providing you momentary comfort when no one else is there, while quietly robbing you of your health. I turned to foods like ice cream, French fries and cakes when stress was unbearable. I had been coaching thousands of people on getting healthy through a health initiative I joined in October of 2011. But, like the fitness coach who needs to lose 30 lbs., just because you "know better" doesn't mean you always "do better." When I was alone and it was just me and my choices, was I choosing life or death? It was only when I was brought to my knees, praying out to God for a second chance that I had to grasp the reality that **"NO FOOD IS WORTH DYING FOR!"** I knew that I had to stop destroying my health with unnatural, inorganic and fake food in order to begin evolving my health with food that yields life instead of death.

The Bible teaches us that a parent must teach by example. God's word encourages children to embrace a father's instruction and a mother's teaching [Proverbs 1:8 NIV]. **As a mother to an amazing son Tarique and now a grandmother to my beautiful granddaughter Anaya, I had two reasons "WHY" I had to make dramatic changes.** I also have grandparents and a mother who gave me the world when my own was falling apart and to whom I will forever be indebted. If I dropped the baton on my health, it wasn't just my life at stake, but the ripple effect of how it could impact my family. This wasn't the first time food had taken control over my life. When I was just 20 years of age, I had emergency surgery and was moments away from death because of my addiction to junk food. I had to let go of the emotional food cravings that were slowly robbing me of my health, energy and vitality. So I ask you...

What is your why? "**W**hat **h**as **y**ou" so consumed that you lose sleep at night? "**W**hat **h**as **y**ou" on your knees praying at 6 am? It could be your children and/or grandchildren, your family and/or spouse, your mother and/or father, your grandmother and/or grandfather. Life is fragile; it could all disappear in an instant. Most take this gift of life for granted. Life on earth is a one-time gift, and you can choose to devolve or evolve your health for pursuing your life's purpose. God blessed you with a physical body that is a magnificent machine designed with an innate ability for healing. This is the only "physical" body you are ever going to have, so you must protect and honor this gift. Beyond your life, you have a responsibility to your children and family. If you die prematurely, you don't just impact your own life, but also change the course of theirs too. Once you identify your WHY, deciding on a healthier lifestyle is the only choice. If you truly make a decision, it is impossible to go back to an unhealthy lifestyle. There is a difference between deciding and trying. Trying is just a polite way of failing. It is imperative you identify your why, as it will keep you focused on the bigger picture.

Describe your why. Also describe an area of your health you would like to improve in the next 28-84 days._____

_____

_____

_____

_____

Make a Decision

At the end of ten days, they [who ate vegetables and drank water] looked healthier and better nourished than any of the people who ate the royal foods.
[Daniel 1:12, 15 NIV]

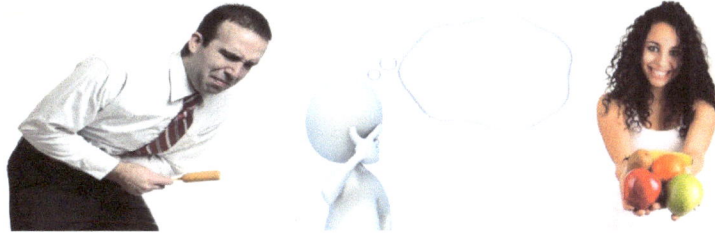

Then they cried to the Lord in their trouble, and God saved them from their distress. God sent out his word and healed them; God rescued them from the grave.
[Psalms 107:19-20 NIV]

Congratulations on making the decision to start PDWP. After your 28-day launch, you either go back to your old lifestyle or complete the remaining 56 days for a total of 84 days. In fact, you might love the results so much that you decide to adopt it permanently as a way of life. To begin, simply fill in your name and start date.

Name _____ **Start (Day 1)** _____

Come let us return to the Lord. God has torn us to pieces but God will heal us; God has injured us but God will bind up our wounds. After two days God will revive us; on the third day God will restore us that we may live in God's presence. Hosea 6:1-2 NIV

Phase One Return (Day 1-28) + Phase Two Revive (Day 29-56) + Phase three Restore (Day 57-84) =
TRANSFORMATION

Return to biblical principles for eating to live. God will **R**evive your heart and mind to **R**estore your spirit, creating a **Transformation** of attitudes and behaviors.

While it is important to launch your journey towards health, to achieve a complete restoration, a total of 84 days is required. Biblically, both 8 and 4 are highly significant numbers. "Proverbs" contains 8 letters and "diet" contains 4 letters. Joined together they signify 12 weeks or 84 days to provide a foundation for improving your health. We divide 84 days into three 28-day phases of achieving your goals with a sense of life's purpose. Three is also an important number. Many significant life-changing events in the Bible happened on the third day. For example, in three days God transforms the life of Jonah, which points to resurrection of Jesus for fulfilling life's eternal purpose.

For as Jonah was three days and three nights in the belly of a huge fish, so the Son of Man will be three days and three nights in the heart of the earth.
[Matthew 12:40 NIV]

Biblically speaking, the number 8 signifies a new beginning, a new birth, and a new order of living with peace, security and prosperity. As a super-abundant number, 8 also represents infinity, empowering you with opportunities to transform your life.

When the whole earth was covered with the flood, it was Noah, "the eighth person" [2 Peter 2:5], who stepped out on to a new earth to commence a new order of things. "Eight souls" [1 Peter 3:20] passed through it with him to the new world.

Biblically speaking, the number 4 signifies praise, balance and division, and invokes the grounded nature of all things. Division signifies the need in our life to simplify goals and projects into smaller units to achieve greater odds for success. The seasons, elements and regions of the earth are all divided by 4. The Bible teaches us to be faithful over a few things and you will be elevated to the next level. Every commitment you make, big or small, elevates you each week until you make it through the complete 84-day program. For this reason PDWP begins with a 28-day launch. The next step (incorporate) will give you the knowledge and tools required for the successful transformation of your mind, body and spirit!

Let food be thy medicine and medicine be thy food.
Hippocrates, the father of medicine (460-357 B.C.)

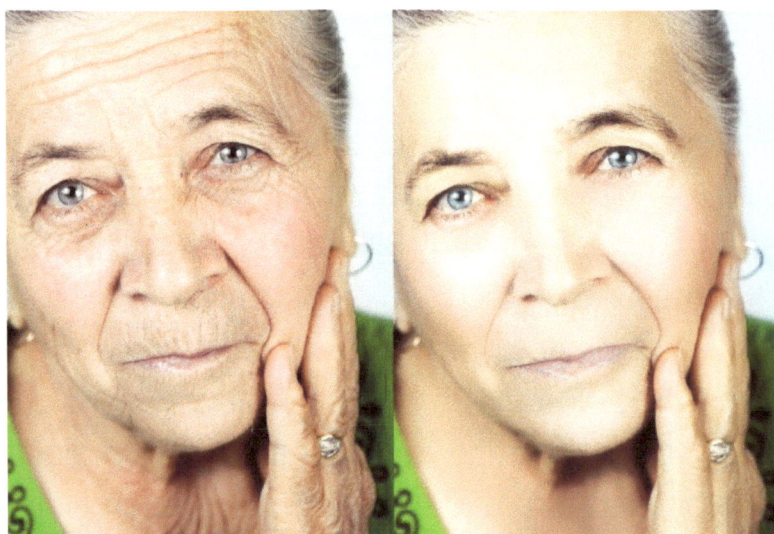

(Step 2) D.I.E.T. = Decide + <u>Incorporate</u> + Educate + Transform

INCORPORATE GOD'S PHARMACY

I give you every seed-bearing plant on the face of the whole earth and every tree that has fruit and seed in it. They will be yours for food. [Genesis 1:29 NIV]

Step 2 of PDWP requires that you incorporate God's pharmacy, which represents natural foods created by God to restore health and vitality. It also contains all the information you need to ensure success. It provides you with the 8 essential resources, biblical proof, scientific evidence and much more. Your Proverbs life coach can also provide you with a customized plan.

8 RESOURCES + 4 STEPS + 84 FOODS + 84 DAYS = TRANSFORMATION

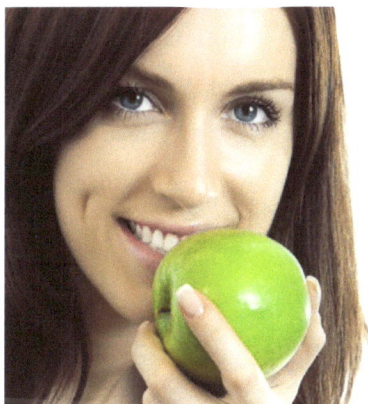

MY PROVERBS LIFE COACH

Name_____

Phone_____

Other _____

8 Resources = <u>P</u>roteins, <u>R</u>ight Carbs, <u>O</u>ils, <u>V</u>ariety, <u>E</u>nzymes, <u>R</u>AW, <u>B</u>alance, <u>S</u>upplements
4 Steps = <u>D</u>ecide + <u>I</u>ncorporate + <u>E</u>ducate + <u>T</u>ransform

The 8 Resources of P.R.O.V.E.R.B.S.

<u>Proteins</u> **(Building Blocks)** Build a brand new body and add muscle and strength.
<u>Right Carbs</u> **(Fuel)** Restore health and beauty with high fiber and low starch.
<u>Oils/Fat</u> **(Nutrient)** Curb cravings; nurture your cells and brain with omega 3.
<u>Variety</u> **(Spice of life)** Enjoy amazing recipes; "meals created for a purpose."
<u>Enzymes</u> **(Digest)** Digest food easier and absorb more nutrients with enzymes.
<u>Raw</u> **(Vitality)** Uncooked food contains life force energy that revitalizes your health.
<u>Balance</u> **(Stability)** Learn the correct ratio of proteins, carbs, fiber and fats.
<u>Supplements</u> **(Replenish)** Boost your immunity, reduce inflammation and more.

Biblical Proof that P.R.O.V.E.R.B.S. D.I.E.T. is the Answer

Wisdom: The ability to discern or judge what is true, right or lasting. *Has not God made foolish the wisdom of the world?* [I Corinthians 1:20 NIV]

After witnessing the premature death of so many who died before their time, I threw myself into discovering why. I read hundreds of publications, articles, scientific reviews, and books and watched countless documentaries. But it was ultimately one book that provided me the biggest clues, and that was the Bible. The book of Proverbs is the book of wisdom. **Proverbs 4:23 NLT tells us, "*Above all else, guard your heart, for it determines the course of your life.*"** In this verse, "heart" refers to one's mind. So, if our mind determines the course of our life, if we do not guard it, disease will occur inside of our body and alter our course forever.

When Solomon refers to "guarding your heart," he means our mind: our thoughts, desires, feelings, actions, behaviors and choices. Our character determines our destiny and it is born out of our inner core. Therefore, "our mind" reflects who we are, not simply our actions and words. Just as our thoughts can cause our physical hearts to harden and allow disease to take over, our spiritual heart can harden as well. We can be faithful believers with positive thoughts who make poor lifestyle decisions regarding food and die prematurely. But, if we want to live out our life's purpose, our prayers must include asking God for the wisdom to make the right choices in all areas of our life. This includes the food we prepare for ourselves and our families.

It is more important to know what sort of person has a disease than to know what sort of disease a person has. – Hippocrates

Solomon also uses the term "course of your life" (which is also referred to as "wellspring" in other versions of the Bible). A course or wellspring is a source through which all things run: love, peace, joy, but also resentment, anger and hatred, and even the food and drinks we consume. **Poor eating habits or negative thoughts and feelings cause our arteries to clog and cut off our flow.** When this happens not only do we become unwell, but we will suffer dire consequences. In fact, the mind is typically the first area impacted by malnutrition. There are over a billion people in the world who are overfed, overweight and malnourished, just like the billion plus who are underfed, underweight and malnourished.

As a man thinketh so is he. – King Solomon

Atherosclerosis is the hardening of the arteries due to accumulated cholesterol plaques and scarring in the artery walls. Hardening of the spiritual heart can also occur.

Arteries are blood vessels that transport oxygen throughout our entire body. They pump blood to our heart, brain, fingers and toes etc. When the inner walls of the arteries are free from plaque, are smooth and haven't hardened from the wrong foods, emotional trauma or negative thoughts, the blood flows freely. **When the blood flow to the heart is blocked it leads to rapid cell death and causes a heart attack.**

PDWP reminds us that we must yield this to a higher power, and use the wisdom given to us by God. There is a weapon bigger than any nuclear bomb, any global warming and any lab-made food, and that is the power of God to bring healing to the people, but it's only if we receive the word in our mind and utilize God's pharmacy. Medication from our doctor was designed for temporary use to save or enhance our life. Many medications are made using natural herbs that have been altered through modern technology. Short-term use of these can be lifesaving; however, long-term use and abuse of medication becomes toxic to our body, especially our liver.

Have you heard the statement, *"I am going to die when 'God' says it is time?"* We were given free will and dominion over the land and were born with the power to choose life or death. **We must not blame our premature death on God.**

Are African American men valued less by God than those of other races? Of course not, but yet they die first. In fact, regardless of race, men die before women across the board. Of all the people who live for more than 100 years, 85% are women. Men are born so strong and genetically nearly perfect, but are still being brought down to their knees, dying faster than women and developing the most aggressive forms of prostate cancer, heart disease, colon cancer, diabetes and strokes.

Does God value people in Mississippi less than people in California? Of course not, but California is near the top of the life expectancy chart while Mississippi is dead last. Mississippi also suffers from some of the nation's highest amounts of diabetes and obesity. Experts predict that by 2030, 67% of people in Mississippi will be obese. If that happens, by this same period close to 100% of people in Mississippi will be overweight.

God doesn't value one group of individuals over the next because every day we wake up with the power to choose life or death; it's our choice. With proper nutrition, utilizing God's pharmacy we can implement changes to prevent metabolic disorders, hormonal balances, thyroid issues, cancer, heart disease and so much more.

The Standard American Diet (S.A.D.) doesn't address the healing mechanisms put in place by God to ensure the survival of the human race. More than 70% of the people we love will DIE prematurely on the American DIE...T. We think day to day, month to month or even moment to moment while God thinks in terms of eternity. Our bodies are magnificent machines, brilliantly designed by God. PDWP addresses the fact that disease occurs when we go against our genetic design. **Genesis 1:26-31 reminds us that God provides us with organic and natural seed-bearing food for everlasting life in fellowship with God and one another into future generations.** Daniel 1:8, 15 explains that Daniel resolved not to defile himself with the royal food and wine and wanted only vegetables and water and as a result looked healthier and better nourished after 10 days. Philippians 4:19 also reminds us that God will supply ALL of our needs, including our food.

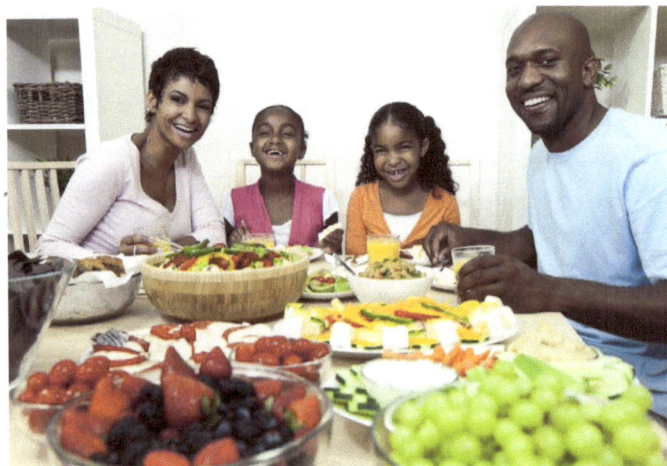

Psalms 107:18 shows that when the people rejected God's organic and natural food and chose unhealthy food, they drew near the gates of death. Now, in modern times, we have repeated history by rejecting the food offered by God for healing and restoration. The consequences we face are much deadlier because not only is our food inorganic and unnatural but it is heavily loaded with chemicals, toxins and even artificial substances, all of which increase death and disease. Humankind has existed for tens of thousands of years in perfect harmony with nature. We have violated the evolutionary chain and are the first group of people to eat food so blatantly disconnected from our roots. We are now consuming processed lab-made food, instead of eating food from nature that grows from the ground or from trees. It has been proven that animals that spend a lifetime on this new artificial diet develop

tumors, heart disease and die prematurely. And yet this type of diet is considered safe for our children to eat and they are now sicker than ever.

Saturated fat, which contributes to heart disease, is found in all animals and is not lab-made. In moderation our bodies utilize fat as a nutrient to supply the cells of our body. Animal protein was considered the superior form because it provides all nine of the essential amino acids. However, overconsumption and the modern practice of overcooking animal protein causes high cholesterol, gout and cancer. Once meat is cooked well done, it loses virtually all nutritional value. Furthermore, it takes an enormous amount of energy for our body to digest cooked meat. God didn't design the practice of cooking meat. Undercooked meat, due to modern agriculture can cause death as well as due to E. Coli and other bacteria found in our meat supply. Irradiation is a process now used to kill these pathogens found in raw meat. While the FDA rules this safe, this is clearly far from God's natural way.

"The beef industry has contributed to more deaths than all of the wars of this century, all natural disasters, and all automobile accidents combined. If beef is your idea of 'real food for real people,' you'd better live real close to a real good hospital." Neal Barnard, MD President, Physicians Committee for Responsible Medicine

In addition to our overconsumption of saturated fat, food scientist intent on improving taste and the shelf life of food have now created trans fats (chemically altered fat) and even in moderation these are lethal and directly linked to heart disease. These are often found in French fries, fried foods, cakes, cookies and other processed foods that line the shelves in grocery stores and restaurants. They have become so problematic that Michelle Obama asked some of the leading grocery stores to remove trans fats from their food supply within the next five years.

Guided by the biblical principles of our loving God, supported by science and experience, PDWP aims to prevent and reverse potential ties of disease and death, and hence empower people to enjoy long-lasting wellness for fulfilling life's purpose. By utilizing natural organic food created by God, miraculous healing occurs, cravings disappear, and weight drops off. This plan is the answer to the prayers of millions of people who want to lose weight and get healthy in the process. This plan is backed by scientific evidence as well as life-saving tools such as the progress report, the formula, nutritional data, important steps, recipes, a grocery list and recommended supplements.

Proverbs Progress Report

Day 1 _____ Weight _____ Hips _____ Waist _____ BMI _____ (Start)

Blood Pressure _____ Blood Glucose_____ Blood Oxygen_____

Day 28_____ Weight _____ Hips _____ Waist _____ BMI _____ (Return)

Blood Pressure _____ Blood Glucose_____ Blood Oxygen_____

Day 56_____ Weight _____ Hips _____ Waist _____ BMI _____ (Revive)

Blood Pressure _____ Blood Glucose_____ Blood Oxygen_____

Day 84_____ Weight _____ Hips _____ Waist _____ BMI _____ (Restore)

Blood Pressure _____ Blood Glucose_____ Blood Oxygen_____

Take a before and after picture. It is also important that you visit your physician prior to beginning PDWP and record your health data. Get checked for vitamin D deficiencies, thyroid, low iodine, and even low glutathione. Low vitamin D levels have been linked to cancer (e.g. prostate) and depression. Calculate your BMI (Body Mass Index) and daily caloric intake for weight loss at www.ProverbsDietOnline.com.

Heart disease risk factors include any of the following: smoking, snoring, waist size greater than 35" for females and 40" for males, diabetes, overweight, physically inactive, family history, insomnia (3 nights or more less of than 6 hours of sleep), resting heart rate higher than 90 beats per minute (normal is 60-80), headaches, high blood pressure and inability to touch your toes (it that signals your arteries might be stiff). **If you have belly fat but are not considered obese, you might have a greater risk factor for heart disease and diabetes than an obese individual.** The waist to hip formula below might save your life. Simply divide your waist measurement by your hip measurement.

WAIST TO HIP FORMULA

Gender	Excellent	Good	Average	At Risk
Females	<0.75	0.75-.79	0.80-0.86	>0.86
Males	<0.85	0.85-0.89	0.90-0.95	>0.95

The Proverbs Formula

(Protein = 20% of Total Daily Calories) For **breakfast** start your day with a liquid protein shake, either whey protein concentrate or hemp. For more protein add low-fat cottage cheese, yogurt or tofu. **Lunchtime** should consist of your largest amount of protein. Choose from whey, hemp, legumes, tofu or an animal source like lean chicken or salmon. **Snack** on low-fat organic plain yogurt or cottage cheese (add berries). During **dinner** utilize only vegetables, beans or grains for protein. **Based on a 2000 calorie diet 20% equals 400 calories (100 grams) of protein.**

(Right Carbs = 40% of Total Daily Calories) Save your carbs for dinner! For **breakfast** avoid fruit, oatmeal or cereals. These items are better suited for dinner because of their high carbs. If you drink the recommended protein shake, it contains grains like oat, millet, buckwheat or quinoa. The only other carbs recommended for breakfast are berries and/or leafy greens, both of which go great in a protein shake. During **lunch** think high fiber carbs like broccoli, celery, and berries etc. This is the perfect time to incorporate green power hour, which is a healthy smoothie with your choice of spinach, kale, celery, carrots, apples and berries. **Snack** on carbs like celery, green apples, carrots and berries. At **dinner** utilize legumes, grains, brown rice, vegetables, starchy vegetables (except white potatoes), root vegetables, and virtually all fruit is fair game for dessert. Strive for at least 40 grams of fiber and less than 25 grams of sugar daily. Fruit has natural sugar, so eat sparingly. For maximum weight loss limit fruit to 2 pieces daily and increase vegetables to 4-6 servings. **Based on a 2,000 calorie diet, 40% equals 800 calories (200 grams) of carbs.**

(Oil/Fat = Up To 40% of Total Daily Calories) During **breakfast**, eat the biggest share of your heart healthy fats like fish oil, flax oil, hemp seeds, chia seeds, ground flaxseeds, and unsweetened almond or peanut butter. Add healthy fat to your protein shake and it will completely curb your appetite for hours. Skip the fat at **lunch** by selecting lean sources of meat or lite tofu. **Snack** on unsalted fats like walnuts, cashews, pistachios, almonds, kale crunch or pumpkin seeds. At **dinner** you should avoid or limit fat, with the exception of coconut oil. **Based on a 2,000 calorie diet, 40% equals 800 calories (88 grams) of fat.** During phase two, fat calories are reduced by half to 20%. During phase 3, or for those with heart disease, daily fat should be 10-15%. Also, if you are taking a vitamin D supplement, it is fat soluble and must be taken with fat in order for your body to properly utilize it.

Nutritional Data

Protein is more than just steak and chicken. Protein is the building block of life, found in every cell essential to living. Good protein builds a strong body (even hair and nails).

Whey Protein Concentrate provides powerful immune enhancing benefits and positive effects on muscle development. The best type of protein for muscle building is luecine, which is available in whey protein. Certain whey products also help stimulate the production of glutathione. Glutathione is naturally contained within our bodies and acts as a buffer for harmful toxins, chemicals and damaged cells. It goes in and absorbs all of the harmful things that can create problems inside of our body. When we don't have enough glutathione we are fortunate to get rid of even one of the harmful invaders. **Most serious illnesses like cancer, diabetes, chronic fatigue, Parkinson's etc. are all associated with low levels of glutathione.**

Hemp seeds contain 21 amino acids, including the 9 essential amino acids your body cannot produce. In fact, just 3 tablespoons yields 10 grams of protein. It contains a high percentage of the simple proteins that strengthen immunity and fend off toxins.

Examples of protein
1 cup of dry beans = 16 grams
3 ounces of meat = 21 grams
1 cup of broccoli = 6 grams
8 ounces of protein shake = 10-16 grams (approx.)
½ cup low-fat cottage cheese = 13 grams

Right Carbs provide fuel for the body. In order to receive the benefits of fuel rather than the typical high carb energy crash, purchase carbs with no added sugar and 1 gram of fiber for every 5 grams of carbs. At dinner a ratio of 1 gram of fiber to 10 grams of carbs is acceptable. **Gluten-free alternatives are also available for those with celiac disease, gluten sensitivity or bloating.** Many gluten-free products are heavily processed, so read the labels.

Carotenoids like carrots, sweet potatoes, tomatoes, apricots and beets are brightly colored and contain lycopene and vitamin A. **A diet rich in lycopene has been proven to prevent the growth of particularly aggressive cancers** and might help reduce the risk of prostate cancer by 45%. The most common cancer among men is prostate cancer, and those with low levels of beta-carotene show a 45% increase risk factor. There are more than 700 carotenoids. Most people are only familiar with a few. **Astaxanthin is from the carotenoid family and is now believed to be the most potent antioxidant nature has to offer.** Learn more on page 32.

Anti-cancer foods like garlic, onions, shallots, leeks and chives can help reduce insulin by regulating blood sugar levels. **These can trigger the death of cancer cells in the colon, breast, lung and prostate.**

Cruciferous vegetables like cabbages, sprouts, broccoli and cauliflower contain anti-cancer molecules and can **reduce the risk of prostate cancer by 41%.** Boiling them destroys these molecules so you should lightly steam, sauté or eat raw.

Sea vegetables (kelp, arame, hiziki, kombu and wakame) and other foods such as cranberries, strawberries, organic yogurt and navy beans contain iodine. The body needs it to make thyroid hormones, which regulate metabolism and other functions. **This deficiency is linked to cancer (breast, prostate, ovarian and endometrial), goiters, heart disease and inflammation.** Even WHO reports show that more than half of Europe and one third of the world (129 countries including the US) have not seen a decline in neonatal mortality in 20 years, and the deficiency also contributes to autism and high cholesterol. Many pregnant women are deficient in iodine, and this can cause a low intelligence quotient [IQ] and learning problems.

Oil/Fat – Omega-3 fatty acids from sources such as flaxseeds, walnuts, chia seeds and hemp seeds are good sources of alphalinolenic acid (ALA). Animal sources of omega 3 like fish oil capsules and salmon contain (DHA) docosahexaenoic acid and [EPA] eicosapentaenoic acid. ALA must be converted into DHA and EPA to provide the full omega 3 health benefits. In most healthy individuals ALA from non-animal sources converts into DHA and EPA. Most diabetics and schizophrenics cannot make this conversion and should take fish oil capsules.

It is estimated by some health experts that more than 90% of the population in the US is deficient in omega 3. The benefits of omega 3 include: helping with rheumatoid arthritis, joint pain, inflammation, prostate cancer, stroke, blood clots, cardiovascular disease, poor circulation, skin disorders, fatigue, schizophrenia, osteoporosis, cognitive decline, systemic lupus erythematous (SLE), menstrual pain, depression, asthma, ADHD, prenatal health, bipolar disorder, reducing blood fat known as triglycerides, and protection against Alzheimer's and dementia.

Other Important Steps

1. **P**artner up – It is easier to lose weight and get healthy when you have accountability partners. Select up to three people who will keep you on track. Accountability Partner(s) 1._____ 2._____ 3._____

2. **Remove** – **Go through your kitchen and eliminate the 8 types of food that contribute to obesity and other health issues:** sugar (high fructose corn syrup, brown sugar and white sugar), artificial substances (aspartame, sucralose, colors, flavors, trans fats, GMOs and MSG), fruit juice, refined flour (including bread and pasta), white rice, corn, white potatoes, and ALL processed junk food. **Note:** While certain types of alcohol offer benefits to reduction of heart disease, it increases risk of breast, throat, esophageal and other cancers.

3. **O**xygenate – You can live weeks without food and days without water. But deprived of oxygen you will die within minutes. People are shallow breathers, so practice deep breathing. Cancer thrives in low oxygen environments. Drink at least 8 glasses (8 ounces each) of water daily to help push toxins out and bring oxygen in. Based on your body weight, activities and other liquids utilized, you might need more or less water per day. Drinking a glass before bedtime might help to prevent a stroke or heart attack; a glass one hour before meals helps you to eat less; and two glasses after waking up can activate your internal organs.

4. **V**isualize – Utilize a vision board to keep track of your goals (your why).

5. **E**xercise – Incorporate running, 10,000 steps daily, zumba, aerobics and/or strength training. Studies show that 2 minutes a day of rebounding (aka mini trampoline) can flush out the lymphatic system, triple white blood count and destroy cancer cells. In *Jumping for Health*, Dr. Morton Walker claims that: "Just 2 minutes of rebounding offers equivalent physiological benefits as 6 minutes of running, 10 minutes of swimming and 22 minutes of walking."

6. **R**est – This is a critical part of the healing and weight loss process. Incorporate 8 hours of sleep every night with optimal sleep hours between 11 p.m.-4 a.m.

7. **B**uy Organic – Apples, grapes, berries and leafy vegetables are more susceptible to pesticides penetrating through the skin. Buy those types of items organic. Fruit like grapefruits and melons you can purchase non-organic.

8. **S**ave Money – Compare prices, order dry goods online, clip coupons, shop on Mondays (for best prices), grow a garden, bring a brown bag lunch, join a wholesale club, and freeze leftovers to make healthy eating affordable.

Recipes - *"Meals Created for a Purpose"*

Variety's the very spice of life that gives it all its flavour. –
William Cowper, English Poet

Variety is the SPICE of life! PDWP defines F.O.O.D. as the **F**lavor **o**f **O**ur **D**estiny. Incorporate delicious recipes that excite the palate and yield long-lasting life. Each meal has been carefully designed to nourish your brain, build a strong body and give you energy and vitality. These are meals created to stop cravings and end the diet rollercoaster forever. This is more of a Proverbs Lifestyle, far removed from your typical diet that requires you to utilize the elusive trait known as "willpower." **When you feed your starving brain, you turn off the out-of-control cravings for life!**

*****SPECIAL IMPORTANT ALERT*****
By replacing processed food with fruit, lean meat, whey protein, vegetables, nuts, seeds, low-fat yogurt and cottage cheese you will **naturally lose weight.** Therefore, eat the same amount of food you normally would during the first two weeks. **If you reduce your caloric intake too quickly, you will lose muscle and end up with more fat and a slower metabolism.** Gradually reduce calories by 10% each week, starting in week 3.

To achieve this, eat smaller portions. To improve your digestive system, chew your food at least 8-10 times before swallowing! Also drink a glass of water one hour before every meal to help control your appetite.

To keep track of proteins, carbs and fats, download the calorie tracker at www.ProverbsDiet.com.
Phase 1 = 20%, 40%, 40% for proteins/carbs/fats
Phase 2 = 20%, 60%, 20% for proteins/carbs/fats
Phase 3 = 15%, 70%, 15% for proteins/carbs/fats

Breakfast – Designed to **nourish your brain w/fat**, most people overeat because their brains are starving! Eat healthy fats, liquid protein and more fiber!

Lunch – This is the time you want to **power up w/protein and greens**. Select leafy greens or high fiber vegetables and lean protein. To accelerate fat burning and curb appetite for hours, adapt the green power hour daily at lunch.

Dinner – This is the time you want to **fuel up w/carbs**. Think of this as a quick refuel after a long day of depleting your body. Load your body with healthy carbs with lots of fiber and phytonutrients. In fact, "Save Your Carbs for Dinner." Source your protein from vegetables or legumes and go low on the fat.

Snacks – This is the time to **curb appetite w/fiber or fat,** so grab high fiber fruits and veggies or good healthy fats like unsalted almonds or walnuts.

Dessert – Done right, an after-dinner dessert should **satisfy the cravings for sweets.** Replace sugar with stevia, lu han guo, evaporated cane juice, or raw honey. Pick desserts like air popped popcorn (non-GMO), seasoning with garlic, Himalayan sea salt, pepper or nutritional yeast.

BREAKFAST

Chocolate Peanut Butter Cup
2 scoops of chocolate whey protein concentrate (or hemp protein)
1 tbsp. Barlean's flax oil and/or ground flaxseed
1 tbsp. raw unsweetened cocoa nibs (see directions)
8 oz. almond or rice milk, unsweetened (or use water)
1 tbsp. raw unsweetened peanut/almond butter (see directions)
1 tbsp. low-fat cottage cheese
3 cubes of ice

Directions: Blend all ingredients. This recipe will curb your appetite and excite your palate. Choose either cocoa nibs or peanut/almond butter, but not both. If you use cocoa nibs, it will taste more like a chocolate chip shake. Flax oil will curb your appetite and flaxseeds add fiber for better elimination. Cocoa nibs provide magnesium and other nutrients. It is best to utilize both flax oil and flaxseed. This makes 1 serving.

Strawberries-N-Cream
2 scoops of vanilla whey protein concentrate (or hemp protein)
1 tbsp. Barlean's flax oil and/or ground flaxseed
½ cup frozen unsweetened strawberries
1 tbsp. low-fat cottage cheese
8 oz. almond or rice milk, unsweetened (or use water)
3 tbsp. ice

Directions: Blend all ingredients. Avoid adding banana during breakfast or lunch until you reach your ideal weight. This makes 1 serving.

Vegetable Omelet (Optional During the Weekend)
8 oz. tofu lite firm (or 4 eggs/egg whites)
3 tbsp. nutritional yeast
¼ red bell pepper

¼ onion
¼ cup of shiitake mushrooms
¼ cup of tomatoes
1 tsp. coconut oil
Himalayan sea salt
cayenne pepper
ground black pepper

Directions: Tofu is a great replacement for eggs or egg whites. Crumble tofu inside a bowl and add vegetables and seasoning. Heat coconut oil over medium heat and then add tofu scramble. If you utilize this option, it is important to drink your protein shake at lunch because you need the liquid protein at least once a day. Remember, whey protein concentrate is recommended for increasing your body's muscle mass and boosting your immune system. This makes 2 servings.

LUNCH

Green Power Hour (Plus Protein Booster)
2 cups of dark green leafy vegetables (kale or spinach)
½ cup of frozen organic berries
½ cup of carrots or celery
1 organic Granny Smith apple
8 oz. of water
2 tbsp. chia or hemp seeds (protein booster)
1 tbsp. spirulina (optional)
3 ice cubes

Directions: Blend all ingredients. **This is the best choice for weight loss because it leaves you full for hours.** Drink approximately 20 ounces. This makes 1 serving.

Green Power Salad (Plus Choice of Protein)
2-3 cups of dark leafy greens
½ cup of tomatoes
¼ cup of carrots
¼ cup of cucumbers
¼ cup of sprouts
3 tbsp. hemp seeds (protein booster)

¼ cup of walnuts or avocado
2 tbsp. nutritional yeast or raw goat cheese
apple cider vinegar
3 oz. of lean chicken, tuna or tofu

Directions: Dice vegetables and mix with leafy greens. Top with protein, nutritional yeast and/or goat cheese crumbled. **This recipe is the best choice for weight maintenance.** Avoid avocado and goat cheese if your goal is weight loss. This makes 1 serving.

Green Power Protein Shake
2 scoops of whey protein concentrate (or hemp protein)
1 cup of dark green leafy vegetables (kale or spinach)
½ cup of frozen organic berries
8 oz. of water
2 tbsp. ground flax seed and/or chia seeds
2 tbsp. low-fat plain yogurt or cottage cheese
3 ice cubes

Directions: Blend all ingredients. **This option works for those looking to lose or maintain weight.** If your goal is weight maintenance leave out chia, greens and berries because the extra fiber will keep you too full to meet daily calories required for weight maintenance. This serves 1.

DINNER

Nachos
15 oz. organic extra-firm tofu (or organic lean ground turkey)
½ cup jalapeno peppers (watch sodium intake)
1 medium onion
3 garlic cloves
garlic powder
1 cup of organic corn and bean salsa
¼ cup of fresh pico de gallo
2 ripe tomatoes
1 cup of red beans
1 pack organic southwest taco seasoning

8 oz. of water
1 avocado
1 tbsp. nutritional yeast
1 cup romaine or kale green leaves

Directions: Dice your onions and garlic and sauté in coconut oil. Mix the organic southwest taco seasoning in water and then crumble tofu and marinate it in the taco seasoning. Add tofu to the pan and continue to sauté on medium heat for 15-20 minutes. Add additional seasonings such as garlic, cayenne pepper and/or crushed red peppers for additional flavor. In a separate pan you can heat the beans for 10 minutes on medium. Make guacamole by combining one large avocado with the fresh pico de gallo. Chop onions, tomatoes and jalapenos for extra topping choices. Layer the bottom with the green leaves, tofu, then beans, guacamole, salsa, onions, tomatoes, and jalapenos. This serves 4-5.

Spicy Marinara
1 onion
1 medium eggplant, sliced into thin strips
1 green bell pepper
4 garlic cloves, crushed
24 oz. marinara sauce (low sodium and no added sugar)
garlic powder
Himalayan sea salt
turmeric
crush red peppers

Directions: Sauté onions over medium heat in coconut oil until transparent and then add garlic. Once garlic is slightly toasted add bell pepper and then eggplant and mushroom. Season with above seasonings of your choice and then add marinara and remaining seasoning. Cooking time is approximately 20 minutes. This serves 4-5.

Three Bean Chili
28 oz. organic whole tomatoes (slice into small chunks)
2 (16) oz. cans organic vegetarian chili (low sodium and no added sugar)
8 oz. organic kidney beans
8 oz. black beans
8 oz. pinto beans, kidney beans & black beans

8 oz. organic extra-firm tofu (or organic lean ground turkey)

2 oz. organic tomato paste

1 cup of chopped eggplant

3 cloves of garlic, chopped or crushed

½ cup of chopped carrots

1 bell pepper

1 large onion

8 oz. of water

2 tbsp. organic southwest taco or chili seasoning

crushed peppers

cayenne pepper

black pepper

turmeric

garlic

lemon zest or juice

Directions: Sautee onions, garlic and bell pepper. After onions are transparent add eggplant. Mix taco or chili seasoning in ¼ cup of water and then marinate the tofu by crumbling tofu inside the mixture. Sprinkle some turmeric on the tofu for coloring and then place tofu in the pan to cook with the vegetables for 10 minutes. Add half of the listed seasonings and then add carrots and tomatoes and cook for about 5 minutes. Next, add the kidney beans, tomato paste, vegetarian chili, water and remaining seasonings. Check the sodium levels on the vegetarian mixture of chili you purchase. If you desire more flavor, add a little lemon zest, extra garlic, cayenne pepper and/or black pepper. Look for low sodium options or make your own chili from scratch. Cook on low for 15-20 minutes or until reach the desired heat. This serves 4-5.

Snacking – Remember that snacks are designed to curb appetite and stop hunger. Daytime snacks can consist of nuts, seeds, apples, kale chips, celery with unsweetened peanut butter.

Desserts – Utilize deserts to satisfy cravings. This is the perfect time to incorporate grapes and bananas. In fact, the Cream-N-Berries recipe, altered for dessert time without the flaxseed and flax oil, can be the perfect way to end your evening. Simply add a half of a banana and even top with low-fat whipped cream. The taste is amazing. Or make it simple and use air-popped popcorn and season with spices, herbs and a very small amount of Himalayan sea salt.

Heart Healthy Cooking Tips

According to *Harvard Health*, salt may be more deadly than you think. While salt is absolutely crucial for the health of certain nerves, muscle fibers and the balance of fluids, most Americans get much more salt than the body requires. The kidneys cannot keep up if there is too much salt in the bloodstream. The heart has to work more and vessels stiffen, which leads to chronic high blood pressure, a risk factor for stroke and heart disease.

More than 70% of the population require restricted amounts of sodium, and actually require far less salt than the recommended daily (dietary) allowance. The elderly and African Americans are especially at risk, along with those who have chronic kidney disease, diabetes or hypertension. **African Americans and people over age 40 should talk with their physician about reducing their daily intake to 1500 mg.** While you have to watch your intake of all sodium, the best is Himalayan sea salt. Just one level teaspoon of table salt and a rounded teaspoon of Himalayan salt is equivalent to 2300 mg.

Replace the extra sodium with fresh herbs and seasonings like apple cider vinegar, basil, garlic, jalapenos, lemons, limes, onions and vegetable broth. Also use dry seasonings like allspice, basil, cumin, cayenne, crushed red pepper, garlic powder, lemon zest, lime zest, onion flakes, oregano, paprika, pepper, thyme and turmeric as well as organic chili and taco seasonings. Some prepackaged seasonings like chili and taco seasoning already contain sodium. Most canned, boxed and jarred foods contain excess sodium. Read labels and select low sodium alternatives.

Turmeric (curcumin) is especially beneficial because it is believed to be useful in increasing glutathione levels. It is an herb extract used in Indian cooking and acts as a potent antioxidant and strong anti-inflammatory. In vitro, it inhibits insulin resistance and cancer cell proliferation and might help improve the effectiveness of chemotherapy. There are so many seasonings to pick from; the key is avoiding MSG and other artificial ingredients.

Now that you are equipped with the nutritional information necessary to navigate through the grocery aisles with less confusion, it's time to go shopping! PDWP provides you with the phase 1 grocery list. For phases 2 and 3 purchase the complete book "P.R.O.V.E.R.B.S. D.I.E.T.: *Wellness for Your Life's Purpose.*"

PHASE ONE GROCERY LIST

*Indicates to purchase organic brands when available. Also purchase non-GMO items; especially food that contains canola oil or corn. **BOLD** indicates to purchase online if not available in stores. Read labels and avoid ingredients from page 22 under step 2 (remove). Visit www.proverbsdiet.com for more information.

Almond Butter*
Almond or Rice Milk, Unsweetened*
Almonds, Raw Unsalted*
Apples, Granny Smith*
Apple Cider Vinegar*
Asparagus Spears
Avocados
Bananas*
Black Eyed Peas*
Beans, All Varieties*
Beets, Red
Blueberries, Unsweetened*
Bread, 100% Whole Grain (avoid added sugar)
Broccoli*
Broth, Vegetable or Chicken*
Brown Rice*
Brussel Sprouts
Butternut Squash*
Cabbage*
Carrots*
Cashews, Raw Unsalted*
Cauliflower
Celery*
Cereal, Gluten-Free Brown Rice*
Cheese, Cheddar or Raw Goat*
Cherries*
Chia Seeds*
Chicken, Breast*
Chili, Vegetarian*
Cocoa Nibs, Unsweetened*
Coconut Oil, Extra Virgin*
Coffee, Healthy
Cottage Cheese, Low-Fat 2%*
Cucumbers*
Edamame*
Eggplant*
Eggs or Egg Whites*
Flaxseed Oil*
Flaxseeds, Golden*

Garlic
Grapefruit
Green Beans*
Greens, All Varieties such as Kale etc.*
Hemp Seeds, Raw Unshelled*
Hummus*
Jalapeno Peppers*
Kale Chips (Watch for Nut Allergy Warning)
Kelp
Lemons
Lime
Mushrooms, Portabella and/or Shiitake*
Nutritional Yeast
Onion, Red, White, Yellow and/or Leeks
Oranges
Pasta Sauce*
Pasta, Penne 100% Whole Grain or Quinoa*
Peanut Butter*
Pineapple Chunks, Unsweetened
Pistachio's, Roasted or Raw Unsalted*
Pumpkin Seeds, Unsalted*
Popcorn, Non-GMO*
Quinoa, Red*
Raspberries, Unsweetened*
Salmon, Red Alaskan or Atlantic
Salsa*
Shallots
Shrimp
Spinach*
Sprouts*
Stevia, Whole Leaf*
Strawberries, Unsweetened*
Sweet Potatoes*
Tea, Green and/or Kumbucha*
Tilapia
Tofu, Lite*
Tomato Sauce*
Tomatoes*
Tortilla Chips, Sprouted NON-GMO*
Tuna, in Water
Turkey, Lean*
Turkey, Lean Ground*
Walnuts, Raw Unsalted*
Whey or Hemp Protein Concentrate
Yogurt, Plain Low-Fat*

Recommended Supplements

Because of the modern society we live in, a healthy diet that incorporates supplements is a necessity if you want to replenish your vitality, increase energy, improve health and prevent disease. Supplements represent highly concentrated antioxidants, vitamins, phytonutrients, minerals, herbs and other botanicals.

ATP

ATP stands for Adenosine Triphosphate. When we are born we produce an abundance of it in our body. Imagine you have millions of dollars in the bank; instead of being proactive and increasing your wealth, you spend every dime and stop producing more. At first it is exciting because you are having the time of your life, but then suddenly you find yourself broke. ATP is the currency of the body that depletes with age. When you have it you have a more youthful appearance, more collagen and a more youthful body. It is the opposite of oxidation, which is when things start to rapidly decay. Without the presence of ATP, oxidation happens because cells have no energy to repair, reproduce or function. When you are under the age of 20, you have an enormous ability to produce this; but as you age, lack of nutrients, oxygen and hydrogen, caused by free radicals, pollution and diet cause you to lose this ability.

Good ATP supplements should increase your body's natural ATP, boost energy and demonstrate results backed by science. Unlike most energy products that utilize artificial sweeteners, flavors, dyes and excessive caffeine, the best choice for an ATP supplement is one that is all natural, provides antioxidant support and contains minimal caffeine through added substances like green tea extract.

Aloe Vera Juice

This wonder tonic has been used for centuries, dating back to the Egyptians who referred to this as the "Plant of Immortality." It is approved by the FDA as a food additive. The following are some of the reported benefits:

*Anti-inflammatory
*Antimicrobial
*Boosts immunity
*Detoxifies the body
*Helps heal cuts, bruises and burns
*Helps support healthy digestive system

*Helps support muscle and joint function
*Improves dermatitis, acne and psoriasis
*Reduces allergens
*Relieves constipation
*Removes harmful bacteria
*Source of essential amino acids and fatty acids
*Source of enzymes, vitamins and minerals

Astaxanthin

This is a nutritional powerhouse from the Xanthophyll family, a subcategory of carotenoid. Carotenoids are produced by plants and animals as a survival mechanism. These are believed to be the most powerful anti-inflammatories in the world. Unlike most antioxidants that oxidize and can only handle one free radical at a time, these handle numerous free radicals and do not oxidize. They go to work on the mitochondria, which is a part of the cells that provide 95% of all energy. Here is a list of some of the reported benefits:

*Alleviates sore joints and muscles
*Anti-aging, reverses external aging and sun damage
*Boosts immune system
*Helps blood pressure
*Helps cardiovascular system
*Improves stamina, muscle function and recovery
*Passes through the blood-brain barrier
*Prevents cataracts, macular degeneration and glaucoma
*Protects eyes
*Protects skin from harsh rays
*Reduces lactic acid
*Strong antioxidant support

Betalains

Chronic inflammation can lead to cancer, cardiovascular disease, arthritis, Alzheimer's, neurological diseases, autoimmune diseases and pulmonary disease. It is estimated that 9 out of 10 people suffer from some sort of discomfort on a regular basis. Betalains are extracted from beets, rainbow chard and the fruit of nopal cactus. It represents a class of red and yellow indole-deprived pigments found in plants. Here are some additional reported benefits:

* Anti-aging
* Anti-inflammatory
* Fights Fatigue
* Fights free radicals
* Fights unhealthy oxidation
* Helps distressed cells
* Improves mental alertness
* Increases energy levels
* Restores body on cellular level
* Supports flexibility

Medicinal Mushrooms

These mushrooms have been used in China for thousands of years for medicinal purposes. The benefits reported from coriolus versicolor known as yun zhi and reishi known as ganoderma are so profound, we suggest you Google the thousands of testimonials. Yun zhi is even used in hospitals in Japan on cancer patients. PDWP makes no medical claims, but provides information so that you and your doctor can conduct your own due diligence.

Medicinal Mushrooms
*Activates antibodies that fight infection
*Aids in stress management
*Anti-tumor
*Boosts immunity
*Increases oxygen utilization
*Protects the body from foreign bacteria
*Reduces insomnia and anxiety

Reishi side effect: Can cause gastrointestinal discomfort. It might have a negative interaction with certain medications.

Probiotics

The human body has trillions of cells, but most of the time people do not think about these cells until they are out of balance. Prebiotics like chicory root are necessary to help probiotics thrive. The following benefits of probiotics have been reported:

* Boosts immunity
* Improves absorption of nutrients
* Defends against harmful bacteria
* Increases good healthy bacteria
* Prevents allergies
* Prevents gastrointestinal illnesses
* Prevents vaginal and urinal infections
* Strengthens digestive system

Wheat Grass

Contains 70% chlorophyll which is the basis of all plant life! Here are some of the reported benefits:

*Aids with digestion
*Detoxifies the body
*Improves blood disorders
*Improves blood sugar
*Increases fertility
*Increases oxygen
*Prevents tooth decay
*Purifies the liver
*Reduces high blood pressure
*Removes heavy metals
*Renews cells and tissues
*Source of enzymes

Other supplements recommended include: mangosteen (improves every organ), goji berries (stimulates human growth hormones naturally), bee propolis (acts as a natural antibiotic), milk thistle (provides liver protection), acai berry (beautifies hair, skin and nails), vitamin D3 (prevents certain cancers and improves mood), and saw palmetto with pumpkin seed oil (helps male prostate issues and slows hair loss).

(Step 3) D.I.E.T. = Decide + Incorporate + <u>Educate</u> + Transform

EDUCATE OTHERS BY SHARING 'GOD'S PROMISE'

Now that you are equipped with the knowledge and improved health, consider the principle that "you reap what you sow," as expressed in the "parable of the sower" in Luke 8:1-8. Let's begin by sharing the "good news" with those you know and meet in your regular way of living. The good news represents the fact that our suffering is over. Luke 8:1-8 also references "The Kingdom of God." The Kingdom of God represents overcoming, eliminating and re-establishing that which your adversary tried to take away. We must share God's promise of abundant life and sow seeds of wellness! **Our decisions impact the next 4 generations, together we can break the generational curse of poor health.**

> Ask: *"Is there any area of your health that you would like to improve?"*
> If they answer, *"Yes,"* you respond, *"Great,"* and tell them to look at the 4-minute video on www.ProverbsDietOnline.com.

This is a simple game of sowing seeds of wellness for improving health. Some will respond no; however you keep on sowing. You will have people who appear excited and committed then fall off track; regardless, you keep on sowing. In the parable, the farmer didn't stop sowing and eventually the seeds fell on fertile ground and the harvest was plentiful. It only takes one seed planted in the right soil (person) to launch a "Wellness Revival" that will sweep the US and then the world.

Life (our physical body) is a "one-time" gift granted from God. We must remind those we care about of this gift and about God's Promise. Imagine every person you talk to represents one seed. But instead of planting hundreds of seeds like the farmer, to help spread the good news of health you need to sow just 12 seeds by giving 12 people a specially designed Proverbs book mark that contains a special seed. Of course you have the option to sow into the lives of dozens or even hundreds of people, but the power of 12 biblically speaking is significant and will eventually help impact the multitudes. Many are called but few are chosen. Some will decide not to take action. However, the farmer kept sowing. And eventually like the farmer, if you continue to sow into others, you will discover at least 3 out of the 12 people are fully committed for long-term wellness for advancing their life's purpose. They will hear the word, retain it and internalize the word and experience abundant health!

One Seed Well Planted Can Save a Nation

But the seed on good soil stands for those with a noble and good heart, who hear the word, retain it, and by persevering produce a crop. [Luke 8:15 NIV]

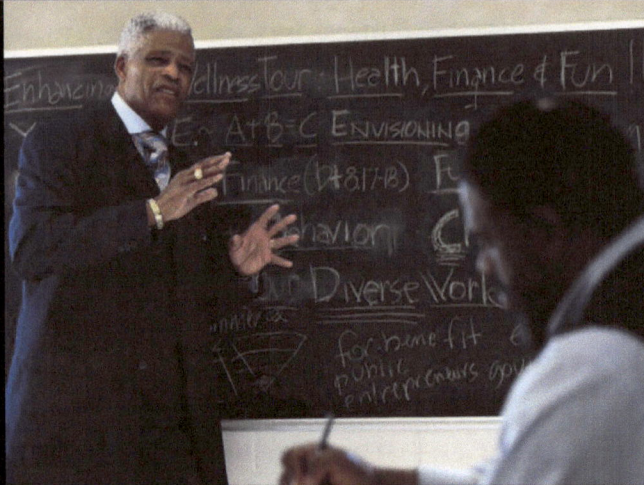

William A. Thurston, Ph.D.
Pictured Standing

You hold the POWER to sow a seed and save a life!

My 12 Seeds Sown
(Give each of the 12 the book mark seed and share the video on www.ProverbsDietOnline.com)

_____   _____   _____

_____   _____   _____

_____   _____   _____

_____   _____   _____

My 3 Seeds that Grew

_____   _____   _____

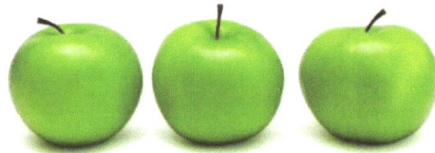

*Individual results will vary. The testimonial on page 37 is not considered typical and should not be used as an indication of what you might experience while on PDWP. Nothing written in this plan should serve as a replacement for medical care. Before undertaking any changes in diet or exercise consult your physician, especially if you are currently on medication or under a doctor's care.

Witnesses of God's Promise

I will bring health and healing to the faithful and let them enjoy abundant life of peace, security and prosperity. [Jeremiah 33:6,9b]

What could have been a tragedy turns into a testimony.

William A. Thurston, Ph.D.
Drops 45 lbs.*
Age 68

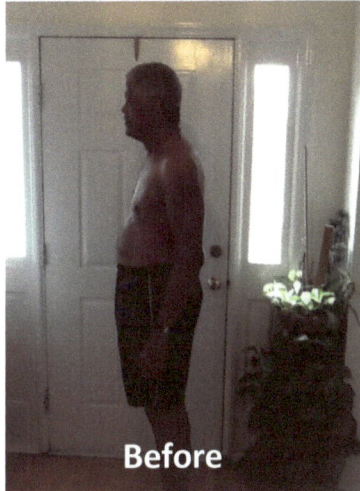

Before

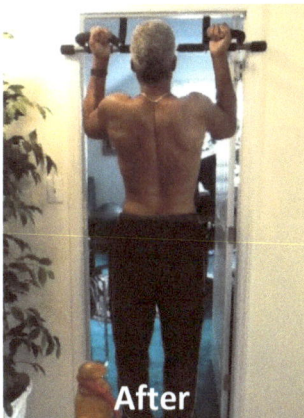

After

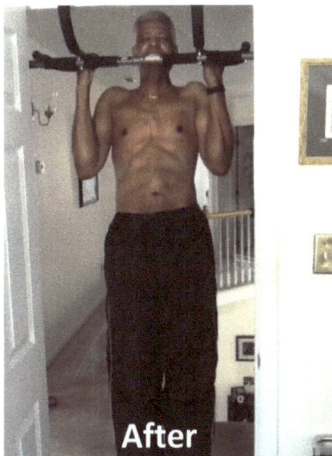

After

I thought I was dying. After getting a clean bill of health from my doctor at age 57, three days later I experienced heart failure after preaching a sermon. God spoke to me on what I thought was my deathbed and revealed to me the consequences of my poor eating habits. I survived quadruple heart by-pass surgery in 2001, but eventually reverted back to these habits. My medical reports of 2011 revealed the resurgence of risk factors for heart and related diseases. Shortly after, I received a phone call from Melissa, who shared a wellness plan with me, and cried out, "We are digging our graves with our fork." **Participating in her programs and incorporating PDWP, I reduced cholesterol from 194 to 147 mg/dl and weight from 235 to 190 lbs.;** eliminated joint inflammation; and increased mental alertness and energy. At 68, I feel more like 38, looking forward to my 6-pack abs by summer of 2013. ☺

Considering my desire to live longer for my family expressed in Proverbs 13:22 to "leave an inheritance" for my family (especially my 7 grandchildren and 2 great-grandchildren), ministries and community based initiatives, I adopted the phase 3 plant-centered diet. I have internalized PDWP, its underlying principles of long-lasting wellness of mind, body and spirit, with time, for fulfilling my life's purpose.

– Raleigh, NC

Witnesses of God's Promise

"For I know the plans I have for you," declares the Lord, "plans to prosper you and not to harm you, plans to give you hope and a future." [Jeremiah 29:11 NIV]

Phyllis N.*

As a baby boomer post menopause, prior to PDWP I struggled for months to lose excess belly fat. Now I am toned, feel fabulous and free from joint discomfort. Feeling lousy does not have to be the norm. Quality of life is important! -Chicago, IL **(Read more on page 42).**

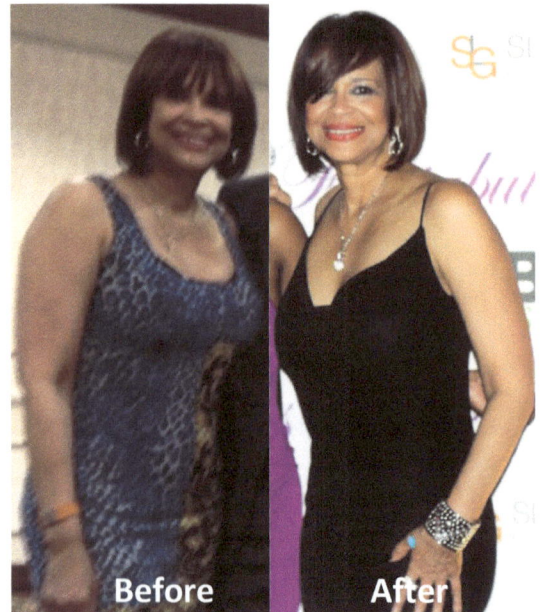

Before   After

Leslie G.*

As a former Vice President for a multi-billion dollar fortune 500 company I've led a hectic life and not always focused on my health. Reaching my 70's I found myself overweight with chronic hip discomfort.

At age 74, I dropped 42 lbs. and no more hip discomfort. My formula to health is whey protein, beet extract and eating healthier according to the principles of PDWP. – Indiana **(Read more on page 43).**

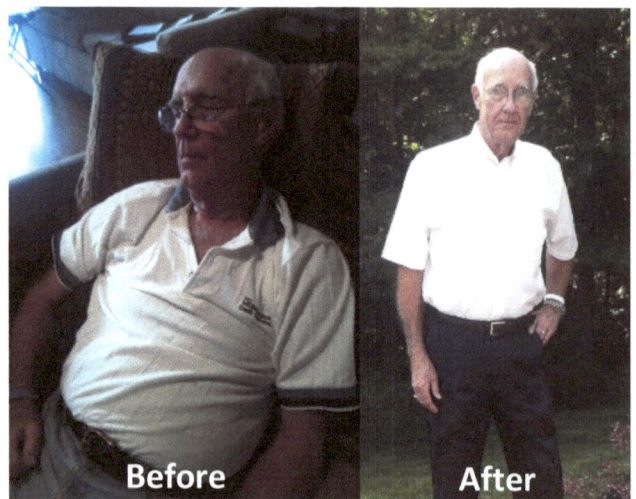

Before   After

*Individual results will vary. These testimonials are not considered typical and should not be used as an indication of what you might experience while on PDWP. Nothing written in this plan should serve as a replacement for medical care. Before undertaking any changes in diet or exercise consult your physician, especially if you are currently on medication or under a doctor's care.

Witnesses of God's Promise

But thanks be to God! He gives us the victory through our Lord Jesus Christ.
[1 Corinthians 15:57 NIV]

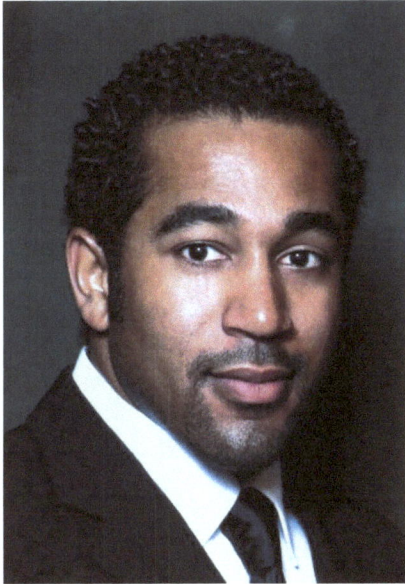

Ian C.*

I have had the unique opportunity and perspective as a Biotech/Pharma Specialty Rep over the past decade to partner with the healthcare community to help ensure that patients stop, look, and listen to solutions that will help improve their lives. At 37, I woke up and discovered that I was on the road to forming multiple risk factors for coronary heart disease (CHD). First, family history of diabetes; second, 25 pounds overweight; and third my waist was almost 2 inches away from 40 inches, which is just as much a risk factor for CHD as smoking. At that point, I prayed and made a commitment to put myself back on a journey for health. Participating in Melissa's training programs I understood the scientific and ethical principles behind the creation of PDWP. Following the nutritional plan and running 5 km every other day, I feel blessed to have been able to lose 30 lbs. and 4 inches off my waist.
– Los Angeles, CA

Despite the billions of dollars spent in research and technology in the area of heart disease, it is still the leading killer of men and now women as well. Read page 16 to learn how to mitigate your risk factors.

Witnesses of God's Promise

The thief comes only to steal and kill and destroy. I came that they may have life and have it abundantly. [John 10:10 ESV]

Bishop Karl Robinson*

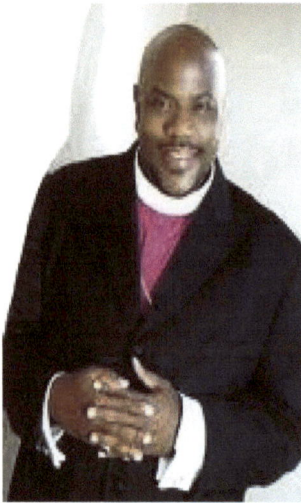

BEFORE

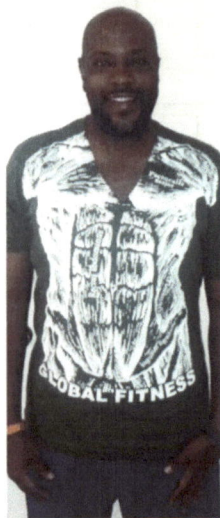

AFTER

After a night of watching basketball and eating pizza, I experienced plaguing symptoms of intense thirst, frequent urination, and lightheadedness. I checked myself into the emergency room and discovered my glucose level was 544 and my blood pressure was 294/197. The lead physician shared with me that I was very sick. I was somewhere between a coma and a stroke. For the next 5 days I was in ICU not even sure if I was going to make it out alive. Once released from the hospital I was prescribed 2 types of insulin and 2 blood pressure medications. After 3 days of shooting myself with insulin, I knew this was not God's will for my life.

*Through many years of trial and error and trying fad diets, I was finally able to rid myself of diabetes, insulin and needles in less than 30 days. Since February 2012, I have been using the whey protein concentrate along with beet extract, which were both advised by my life coach. **Not only have I lost over 100 lbs., but I have also reversed type II diabetes.***

Witnesses of God's Promise

My children pay attention to what I say. Listen closely to my words. Don't lose sight of them. Let them penetrate deep into your heart, for they bring life to those who find them, and healing to their whole body. [Proverbs 4:20-22 NLT]

*****************Dr. Susan H., DDS, Chicago, IL*****************

Despite the fact that I was very active, participating in aerobic/strengthening exercises (Zumba and weight lifting), I reached a plateau. However, I started PDWP and changed my eating habits by replacing some of my normal snacks with unsalted raw almonds. I reduced my meat consumption to 3-4 times a week, adding mostly salmon or lean chicken. By getting most of my fat from omega-3 sources, I experienced a dramatic weight loss. On December 9th I weighed in at 178 lbs.; on December 16th 173.4 lbs.; and 166.4 lbs. by Christmas Day. This was the lightest I had been in years. Even after I fell off the proverbial diet cliff during the holiday, my fat burning process that had been ignited by these new changes continued. I had given up hope after years of failed weight loss programs and finally found a way of life that is simplistic even with a busy schedule. Sometimes we all need that extra push to realize we are going downhill fast with blinders leaving our destiny in the hands of others. I am thankful that this plan helped me to restore my self-image and made my life simpler.

*****************Nettie J., Pastor, Detroit, MI*****************

When I started this journey, I had no idea it would change my life forever. I had some real challenges in the beginning and I had to work through them. On November 26, 2012, less than 5 weeks ago, I was 202 lbs., on blood pressure medication and not feeling good about myself. I am now down to 194 lbs., feeling good about myself and off blood pressure medication. My 66th birthday is just around the corner and I love this life! Thank you Melissa for your obedience to God; because of that many lives will be changed and I am glad to be in the number. As I continue this journey, God has given me a book to write as well. I look forward to seeing this program transform lives on a daily basis.

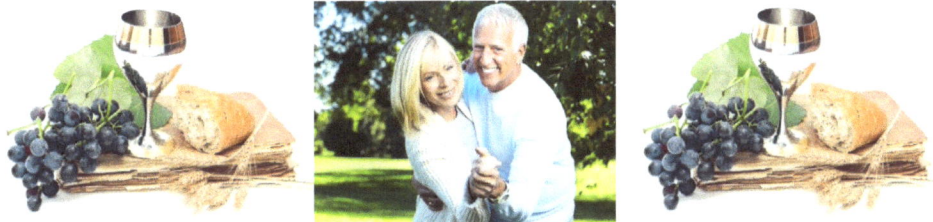

Witnesses of God's Promise

*********************Kathy W., Columbia SC*********************

I lost 8 pounds and reduced ½ inch off my arms, waist and thighs in 5 weeks on PDWP. My cholesterol and blood pressure also improved significantly. I simply add the green leafy vegetables, chia and/or ground flaxseed to my morning protein shake regimen and now my elimination is better than ever. I have lots of energy, and the added fiber keeps me full for hours. This is a lifestyle change that was much needed!

*********************Linda S., Chicago, IL*********************

My physician informed me that I was "pre-Diabetic." In between visits, I found myself in a dangerous situation because my blood sugar was going up instead of down. When I learned about PDWP, I was desperate to get my numbers under control. After two weeks on the plan, my blood sugar dropped from the 170s/160s to the 120s/110s. My skin is glowing and my energy is through the roof. It's also hard to believe that I lost more than 2½ inches off my waist and hips. When my friends saw the new me at Christmas, they could hardly believe my transformation. I love to snack so the fact that this has also helped me to get my cravings under control is truly a God send.

*********************Phyllis N. Chicago, IL*********************

When Melissa shared with me PDWP in October 2012, I started on it immediately. I knew it was what my body needed. Post menopause my body seemed to have a mind of its own and I was bloating at the drop of a hat. Ladies, can you relate? I was working out several times a week, but couldn't drop the extra 5 lbs. that I needed to lose in order to reach my ideal weight. I had excess belly fat under the breast area and rolls in places that at one time were toned. Forty years prior, it took me just 30 days to reach my pre-pregnancy weight after giving birth to my son Torrie. The health benefits of live raw food, kumbucha tea and enzymes are extraordinary. My midsection vanished, my stomach muscles toned, the inflammation in my knee disappeared and I am at my ideal weight. Even my hair, skin, teeth, energy, mobility and mental clarity have all improved.

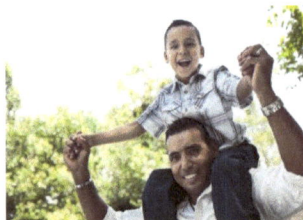

Witnesses of God's Promise

*********************Leslie G., Indiana *********************

At 73 years old, I found myself with limited mobility and pain due to my hip. I was also 42 lbs. overweight. Fortunately, a friend of mine contacted me a year ago and introduced me to Melissa and she shared with me the concept of an 84-day health challenge. In that time, I lost 42 lbs. and have not put it back on. I have eliminated all my prior medications for cholesterol and acid reflux. Now with my doctor's approval, I am completely medicine free. I start my day with the beet-based extract called Betalain and it allows me to move and do my daily activities without any discomfort. My wife is a nurse, so in participating in Melissa's training programs we understood the scientific principles behind the development of PDWP. I have been empowered with a system that is simple and focused providing me with the right nutrition that allows me to keep my now 74-year-old body in a 33 pant size and weight at 164 lbs.

********************Larease R., Atlanta, GA********************

I have always been passionate about supplements that help me feel and look good. I turned 50 in 2012 and people mistake me for someone 20 years younger. I utilize the supplements highlighted in PDWP as a part of my anti-aging regimen. I love the betalains, astaxanthin and enzymes. I have a four-year-old daughter and the energy required to keep up with her is intense. Supplements and healthy eating is the key.

*******************Karen S., Retired, Maryland*****************

When I started the plan, I had no idea at age 67 I would become so concerned about my health. I began on November 26, 2012 with 10 lbs. to lose and within 5 weeks dropped 5 lbs. The timing of this was God sent. My family was devastated when we learned that my 61-year-old brother who had no health issues was diagnosed with stomach cancer and given 6 to 8 months to live. He went home to be with the Lord on December 12, 2012. This loss to my family has given me a greater mission to be healthy and to help others do the same thing. Thank you for obeying God and giving me such a great opportunity. The weight continues to drop. PDWP is a true blessing!

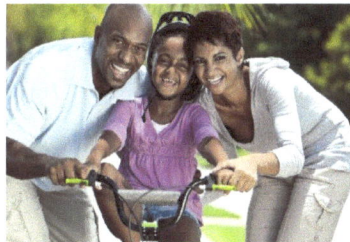

Witnesses of God's Promise

*********************Bridgett B., Atlanta, GA*********************
I am normally plagued with 2 to 3 severe migraines per month, but have not experienced one during the last 30 days since starting PDWP. In this same period, I've lost 5 lbs. and ½ inch off my waist. This is huge for me because normally I lose weight and gain it right back due to fluid retention from a heart condition. So far, the 5 lbs. is staying off and I finally feel like I can reach my ideal weight and stay there. This is truly the best that I have felt in years. Every day I'm experiencing an abundance of natural energy whereas before I use to experience daily fatigue. I'm sleeping much better at night and have no problems getting up in the mornings. Because of the new energy that I have, I'm now able to exercise daily and consistently – something that I haven't been able to do in years. I actually look forward to exercising every day. This plan is the missing piece to my health puzzle. I'm so excited!

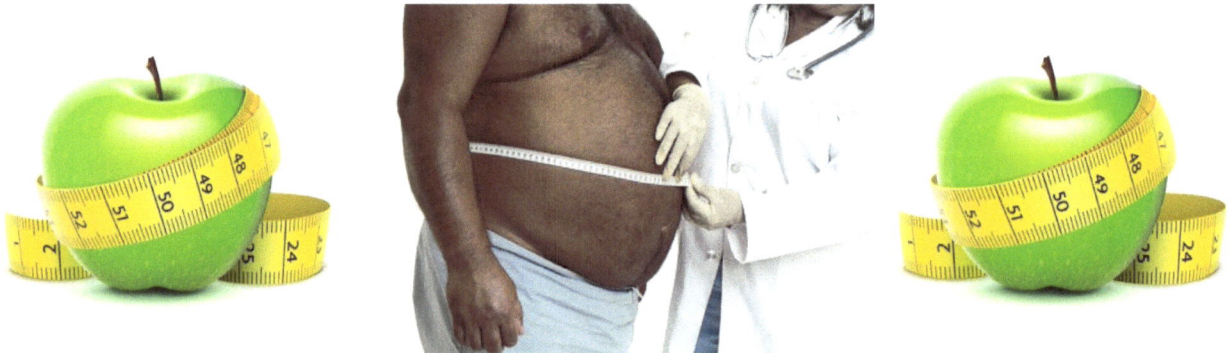

Take the Proverbs Wellness Challenge and email your 28-day and/or 84-day results to support@proverbsdiet.com.

Also **SAVE YOUR RECEIPT!** The purchase of PDWP includes: one FREE member activation to www.ProverbsDietOnline.com to the value of $28.84! This makes PDWP virtually free! In addition to FREE activation of your member account, for a limited time gain complimentary access to more recipes, an online support social community, and the calorie tracker. Register with reference code 12841201. We also offer a complete online coaching system and a "VIP Wellness or Weight Loss Pass" for just $1.84 per week.

*Individual results will vary. These testimonials are not considered typical and should not be used as an indication of what you might experience while on PDWP. Nothing written in this plan should serve as a replacement for medical care. Before undertaking any changes in diet or exercise consult your physician, especially if you are currently on medication or under a doctor's care.

(Step 4) D.I.E.T. = Decide + Incorporate + Educate + <u>Transform</u>
TRANSFORM TO FULFILL 'GOD'S PURPOSE'

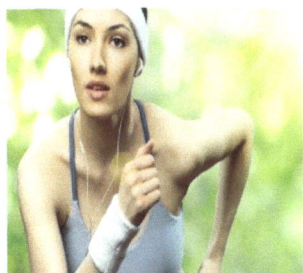

Do not conform any longer to the pattern of this world but be transformed by the renewing of your mind. Then you will be able to test and approve what God's will is – God's good, pleasing and perfect will. **[Romans 12:2 NIV]**

If you **D**ecide, **I**ncorporate, **E**ducate but fail to transform, you ultimately DIE prematurely like millions of others. This fourth step is critical because it represents the internalizing of the 8 resources and making PDWP a way of life. When you faithfully embrace the plan over a 28-day period you earn your promotion to the next level, which is another 28 days. Eventually you will complete the full 84-days and experience a physical, mental and spiritual breakthrough as God transforms you.

God Will Move the Heaven and Earth

Billions of people will live and die and not hear this message, a message that holds the key to healing our children, our families and our community. You had a better chance of playing your odds on the mega lottery and winning than reading PDWP, a plan that holds wisdom that is more valuable than money and material things. The Bible reminds us that a fool and his or her money will soon part. So anyone can be blessed with money or good health. But it is the wise person that holds the secret to recreating both over and over again. Would you rather be blessed with perfect health and a bank account with millions, and be a fool with no skill on how to maintain either; or would you would you rather be in poor health and destitute with an infinite wisdom on reversing both? Because the odds are so small, it is no accident that you are reading this. **God has a will so strong for your life that the Heavens and Earth have moved to ensure you incorporated wellness for your life's purpose.** Your life has a story that needs to be told. When you share that message you unlock the potential for true healing. First you heal yourself and when others realize they are not alone in their struggles your story will heal your family, your friends, your neighbors, your community and perhaps even people around the world.

If you have also purchased PD and completed the entire 84 days, congratulations! We recommend you start an on-going participation in self-transformative programs of wellness advancing life's purpose, glorifying God!

If you or a loved one is battling a chronic disease, "P.R.O.V.E.R.B.S. D.I.E.T.: *Cure*" is the third book and will be available in spring 2013. It provides a daily prayer, meditation, exercise and more supplements and foods to restore health and reverse disease. We must remember Romans 8:28 NIV that reminds us all things God works for the good of those who love him, who have been called according to his purpose. Your purpose manifested before you were born. **Discover what that is, and with your newfound wellness, go fulfill it.**

Describe your life's purpose._____

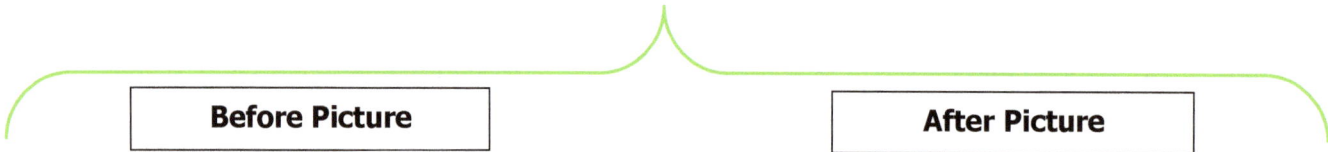

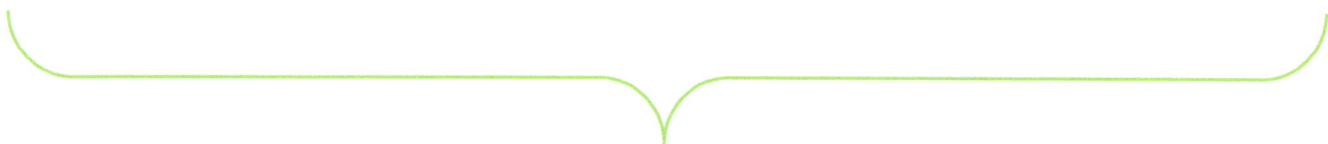

_____

_____

_____.

Before Picture   **After Picture**

References

The following books were most helpful. I recommend you obtain them for your personal library.

The Bible: King James Version, New International Version, English Standard Version and New Living Translation

Campbell, T.C. & Campbell, T.M. (2006). *The China Study*. Dallas, TX: Benbella Diamond.

Fuhrman, J. (2003). *Eat to Live*. New York: Little Brown.

Schlosser, E. (2004). *Fast Food Nation: The Dark Side of the All-American Meal*. New York: Harper Perennial.

Robbins, John (2010). *The Food Revolution: How Your Diet Can Help Save Your Life and Our World*, 10th Anniversary Edition.

Zenn, J.M. (2012). *The Self Health Revolution*.

Calabrese, K. (2011). *Soak Your Nuts: Cleansing with Karyn*.

Kenney, M. (2008). Every Day Raw.

Snyder, C.N.K. (2011). *The Beauty Detox Solution*.

Rose, N. (2007). *Raw Food Life Force Energy: Enter A Totally New Stratosphere of Weight Loss, Beauty, and Health*.

Atkins, R. (2002). *Dr. Atkins New Diet Revolution: Completely Updated! The Must Have New Edition*.

Esselstyn, M.D. & Caldwell B. (2008). *Prevent and Reverse Heart Disease, The Revolutionary, Scientifically Proven Nutrition-Based Cure*.

Bohager, Tom (2006). *Enzymes: What the Experts Know*.

Walker, Morton, M.D. (2005). *Jumping for Health: A Guide to Rebounding Aerobics*

Great Documentaries

Hoffman John & Nevins Sheila (2012). HBO: The Weight of the Nation Part I, II, III and IV

Cross Joe & Kurt Engfehr (2010). Fat, Sick & Nearly Dead

Coloquhoun James (2008). Food Matters

Great Websites

www.FDA.gov

www.health.harvard.edu

www.cdc.gov

www.diabetes.org

www.heart.org

www.cancer.org

Articles

"Rethinking the Meat-Guzzler," Mark Bittman, *New York Times*, January 27, 2008

http://www.nytimes.com/2008/01/27/weekinreview/27bittman.html?pagewanted=all&_r=0

http://men.webmd.com/prostate-enlargement-bph/features/enlarged-prostate-bph-complex-problem?page=3

"These top nutritional performers can transform your diet and possibly your life," Carol Ness, *San Francisco Chronicle*, Wednesday January 4, 2006

http://www.sfgate.com/food/article/THE-POWER-OF-SUPER-FOODS-These-10-top-2544142.php#photo-2681489

http://articles.mercola.com/sites/articles/archive/2010/04/10/can-you-use-food-to-increase-glutathione-instead-of-supplements.aspx

http://www.heart.org/HEARTORG/GettingHealthy/FatsAndOils/Fats101/TransFats_UCM_301120_Article.jsp

http://healthliteracy.worlded.org/docs/tobacco/Unit1/2history_of.html

http://www.heart.org/HEARTORG/GettingHealthy/FatsAndOils/Fats101/Trans-Fats_UCM_301120_Article.jsp

http://www.webmd.com/healthy-aging/omega-3-fatty-acids-fact-sheet

http://healthland.time.com/2012/10/01/guide-the-31-healthiest-foods-of-all-time-with-recipes/slide/blueberries/

http://articles.mercola.com/sites/articles/archive/2012/11/14/waist-size-matters.aspx

About the Author and Co-Creator

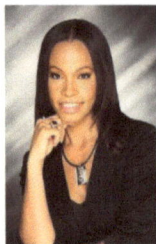

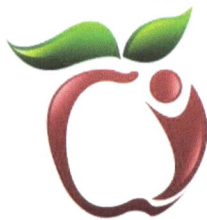

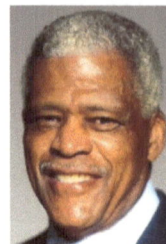

Written by
Melissa A. Boston

Retiring seven years ago from corporate America at the age of 33, as a single mom, she has led the way for women, especially single moms everywhere, who desire time freedom. As Co-founder and Chairlady of the Board of the Ladies of Team Vision, Melissa built an international sales team of 8,000 people in Canada, Bermuda and the United States. Featured on the cover of magazines, on radio shows and even television shows, she is a trailblazer and visionary. Melissa has co-authored three books and does empowering and motivational training in the USA and internationally, in Bermuda, Germany, Mexico, Canada and Bahamas.

In 2006 she achieved the rank of National Sales Director for a network marketing company that grossed over $1 Billion in sales. For her sales performance, innovation and leadership she was honored as MVP in 2011 and selected as one of eight seated members on the National Advisory Council known as the "Super Eight." She walked away from a multiple six-figure income to inspire people to live healthier in the wellness industry.

In 2012 she began writing the book "P.R.O.V.E.R.B.S. D.I.E.T.: *Wellness for your life's purpose"* available March 2013. After working closely with one of her mentors Dr. William A. Thurston, they collaborated and created PDWP.

Today, she is CEO of Proverbs Lifestyle Partners, LLC, a company that offers support, coaching and education to individuals and groups on how to create wellness for their life's purpose. In addition, she was elected to the executive leadership council for one of her affiliates, a network marketing company where she achieved Diamond status. They are an international biotechnology wellness company with over $40,000,000.00 invested in discovering ways to improve the health of the world.

Supplement by and Co-Creator
Rev. William A. Thurston, Ph.D.

Dr. Thurston is a Professor in Shaw University's Department of Religion and Philosophy in Raleigh, NC, serving as department chair for 18 years. Dr. Thurston graduated from the University of Illinois with a Bachelor of Architecture in Design. He also earned both the Master of Divinity (magna cum laude) and the Doctor of Philosophy in Ethics and Society from Emory University in Atlanta, Ga. Prior to his present academic appointment, Dr. Thurston served as professor of Religion and Philosophy and coordinator of Chapel Worship at Shaw University. He has also taught at Columbia Theological Seminary, Atlanta University and Clark College.

Dr. Thurston served as the national director of the Rev. Jesse L. Jackson's Operation PUSH.

As an architect and planner, Dr. Thurston directed redevelopment plans in the U.S. and the Third World.

Internationally, Dr. Thurston is exploring partnerships to prepare leaders and managers for community and civic revitalization in the Americas.

Dr. Thurston and his wife, Gayle, are co-founders of Enhancing Your Life Global: Health, Finance and Fun and host face-to-face and teleconference conversations weekly on "Strengthening Your Spirit," Feeding Your Faith," and "Building Your Biz."

IT IS TIME FOR P.R.O.V.E.R.B.S. D.I.E.T.

The Bible teaches us that a parent must teach by example **[Proverbs 1:8 NIV].** Despite these instructions from God, the people of the US have already given birth to the first generation of children whose life expectancy is ten years shorter than their parents. One out of 3 children born in the US after the year 2000 will face diabetes in their life, one out of 2 if the child is African American or Latino. Spiritually, mentally and physically we are under attack and dying.

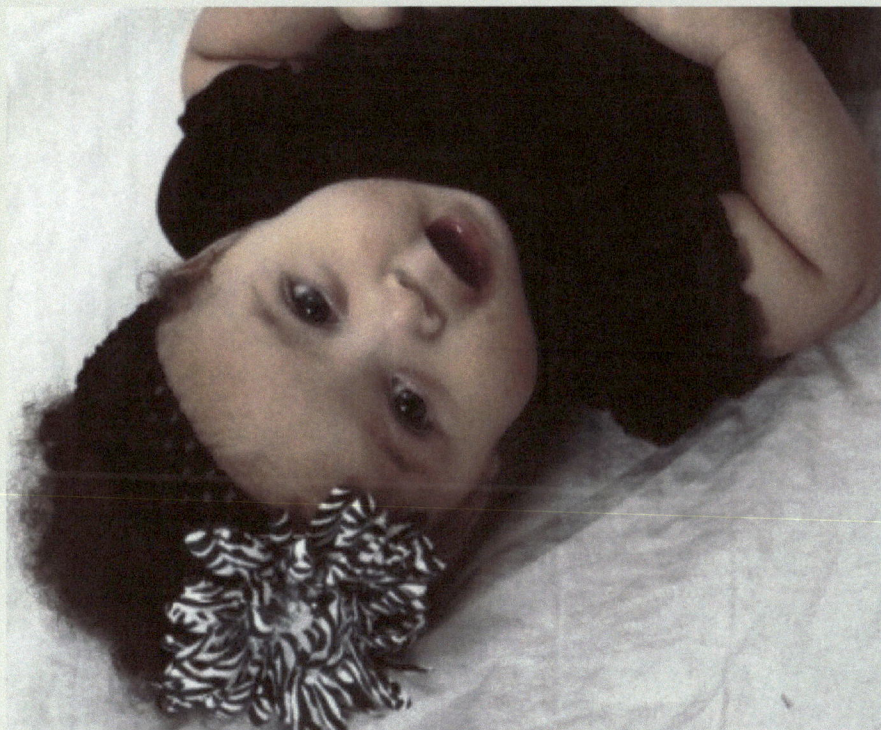

"I dedicate this to my granddaughter Anaya, my son Tarique, my nephew Donovan, my mother Charlotte, my grandparents Margaret and Melvin, my dearest friends Mekalia and Larease, and to your children and our future generations."
Melissa Boston

Let this be written for a future generation, that a people not yet created may praise the LORD. [Psalms 102:18 NIV]

Luke 10:2 NIV reminds us that the Harvest is plentiful, but the workers are few. To reap the Harvest of abundant health, we must sow seeds of wellness into the lives of others by launching a "Wellness Revival."

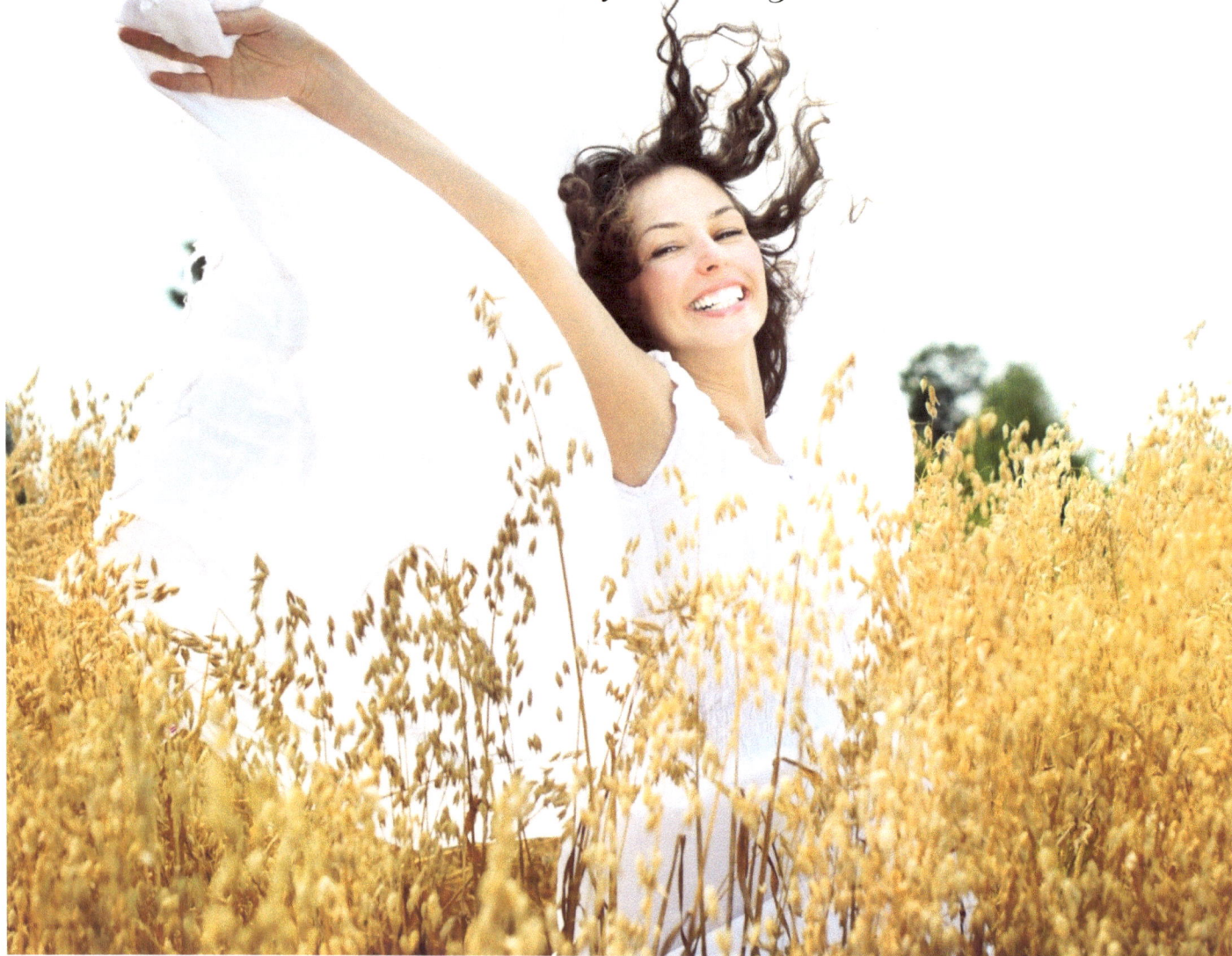

"I truly believe that this project was inspired and given to a 'Brilliant Mind' and one of the most committed and hardworking people I have ever known, Melissa Boston. I believe that if one acknowledges God for direction, God will lead you in places you couldn't imagine you could go. This plan was put together so strategically, carefully, and prayerfully, that those who follow it will be blessed. This is one of the most exciting and beneficial things I have ever done. Melissa, I thank you for giving yourself to be used by God to help other people live." **- Jacquelyne Underwood, Registered Nurse**

"If you only read one weight loss book in your lifetime, **this is the MUST READ book.** It goes beyond weight loss as it addresses mind, body and spirit. As a nutritionist, I was already near my ideal weight but desired to lose a few inches around my midsection. In less than 4 weeks I lost 4 lbs. and 3 inches off my waist." **- Patrice Hughes, Nutritionist**

www.ingramcontent.com/pod-product-compliance
Lightning Source LLC
Chambersburg PA
CDIIW0008002.70120
4192/CB00002B/73